Primer of Geriatric Urology

Thomas J. Guzzo • George W. Drach
Alan J. Wein
Editors

Primer of Geriatric Urology

Consulting Editor
Mary Ann Forciea, MD, FACP
Division of Geriatric Medicine, Department of Medicine
University of Pennsylvania Health System
Philadelphia, PA, USA

Springer   2013

Editors
Thomas J. Guzzo, MD, MPH
Department of Surgery, Division of Urology
Perelman Center for Advanced Medicine
Hospital of the University of Pennsylvania
Philadelphia, PA, USA

George W. Drach, MD
Department of Surgery
Perelman Center for Advanced Medicine
Hospital of the University of Pennsylvania
Philadelphia, PA, USA

Alan J. Wein, MD, FACS, PhD(hon)
Division of Urology
Perelman Center for Advanced Medicine
Hospital of the University of Pennsylvania
Philadelphia, PA, USA

ISBN 978-1-4614-4772-6   ISBN 978-1-4614-4773-3 (eBook)
DOI 10.1007/978-1-4614-4773-3
Springer New York Heidelberg Dordrecht London

Library of Congress Control Number: 2012948766

Springer is part of Springer Science+Business Media (www.springer.com)

Preface

The American population over the age of 65 (the Medicare Population) will grow greatly in the next two decades. The US Census Bureau has estimated that by 2030, 20 % (approximately 72 million people) of the US population will be in this group. Currently one in every ten individuals in the world is over 60 years of age; by 2050 this number will double to 1 in 5. Additionally, due to improvements in medical care, elderly individuals are living longer. In 2004, the median life expectancy for an individual reaching age 65 reached 17.1 years and at age 75, 10.7 years. While many health care specialists will feel the impact of this growing elderly population, few will be more affected than those in the field of urology. Many urologic disorders have an increased prevalence among the elderly: nearly 50 % of outpatients and over 60 % of surgical/procedural patients encountered in US urologic practice are over the age of 65 years.

As medical students on our pediatric rotations, we learn early on that children are not "little adults." The obvious wisdom of this saying is that pediatric patients have a unique physiology and pathophysiology that is not necessarily transferable from what we learn on the adult wards. One can also say the same for our geriatric patient population. Borrowing this phrase from our pediatric colleagues, it is not just as simple as "they are older adults." The elderly urology patient merits special assessment on several fronts. Many nonoperative urologic conditions (such as lower urinary tract symptoms) are treated with medications which can affect cognition and/or interact with other daily medications. Urinary issues, such as incontinence or frequency, can lead to significant morbidity in the functionally impaired, leading to falls. Surgical intervention is common for urologic disease, both oncologic and benign, and must be carefully considered in the geriatric patient.

Our text is intended to provide a review of the demographics of our aging urologic population and their unique needs. We review medical issues particular to the elderly patient that must be considered in the initial evaluation of the aging patient, and follow this with practical suggestions in development of the management plan, whether by medication or invasive procedure. Common complications (and their management) encountered in the treatment of elderly inpatients are also covered. Important aspects of continuity of care are also included, such as the appropriate use of adjunctive services and the urologic aspects of nursing home care. Finally, specific urologic disease processes in the elderly population are reviewed including urologic oncology, lower urinary tract symptoms, and sexual dysfunction.

We believe this book will be useful to anyone who is involved in the care of geriatric patients including medical students, residents, general practitioners, internists, and urologists. This book is not intended to be an exhaustive review of either urology or geriatrics; but rather an easy to use, practical and rationale guide to common urologic management problems in the geriatric population. The chapters are purposefully concise so that health care providers can use the information contained within the book "on the fly"; either on rounds or while seeing patients in the office. It is our hope that this book will aid the reader to better address some of the unique needs of this growing patient population.

Philadelphia, PA, USA   Thomas J. Guzzo

Contents

Contributors

George W. Drach, MD Department of Surgery, Perelman Center for Advanced Medicine, Hospital of the University of Pennsylvania, Philadelphia, PA, USA

Mary Ann Forciea, MD, FACP Division of Geriatric Medicine, Department of Medicine, University of Pennsylvania Health System, Philadelphia, PA, USA

Thomas J. Guzzo, MD, MPH Department of Surgery, Division of Urology, Perelman Center for Advanced Medicine, Hospital of the University of Pennsylvania, Philadelphia, PA, USA

Andrew M. Harris, MD Department of Urology, Hospital of the University of Pennsylvania, Philadelphia, PA, USA

William I. Jaffe, MD Department of Surgery, Division of Urology, Penn Presbyterian Hospital, Philadelphia, PA, USA

Sanjay Kasturi, MD Resident of Urology, Hospital of the University of Pennsylvania, Philadelphia, PA, USA

Eugene J. Pietzak, MD Department of Surgery, Division of Urology, Perelman Center for Advanced Medicine, Hospital of the University of Pennsylvania, Philadelphia, PA, USA

Matthew J. Resnick, MD Department of Urologic Surgery, Vanderbilt University Medical Center, Nashville, TN, USA

Edna P. Schwab, MD Department of Medicine, Division of Geriatrics, Hospital of the University of Pennsylvania, Philadelphia Veterans Administration Medical Center, Philadelphia, PA, USA

Allen D. Seftel, MD Department of Surgery, Division of Urology, Cooper Medical School of Rowan University, Camden, NJ, USA

Ariana L. Smith, MD Department of Urology, Hospital of the University of Pennsylvania and Pennsylvania Hospital, Philadelphia, PA, USA

Daniel Su, MD Department of Surgery, Division of Urology, UMDNJ-Robert Wood Johnson Medical School, New Brunswick, NJ, USA

Alan J. Wein, MD, FACS, PhD(hon) Division of Urology, Perelman Center for Advanced Medicine, Hospital of the University of Pennsylvania, Philadelphia, PA, USA

Philip T. Zhao, MD Department of Surgery, Division of Urology, UMDNJ-Robert Wood Johnson Medical School, New Brunswick, NJ, USA

Chapter 1
Introduction: Aging

George W. Drach

We created this text for you, the urologic resident, practicing urologist and urologic surgeon, so that you would encounter fewer troubles as you care for your elderly patients. We know that in many instances you rely on other physicians or medical personnel to assist you in this geriatric care, but we believe that if you can increase your level of knowledge in evaluation and management of the older patient slightly at the time of your first encounter that you will obtain a smoother course throughout the duration of subsequent management and care of your patient. In addition to this text, a compact major source of reference material regarding geriatric care by specialists other than geriatricians can be found in the manual: "Geriatrics at Your Fingertips" hereafter referred to as GAYF. It is published by the American Geriatrics Society and can be accessed at http:\\www.geriatricsatyourfingertips.org [1].

Demography in the USA

If you treat mostly adult patients, look into your waiting room one day and you will see a large number of gray-haired patients. Urologists see a larger percentage of older persons in their offices than other surgical specialists such as general surgeons, orthopedists, and otolaryngologists (Table 1.1). Only Ophthalmologists see more elderly outpatients and then only by a small margin. Another way to look at the relative activities of surgical specialties is to observe the total number of Medicare patients served in 1 year (Fig. 1.1). In-hospital surgical intervention by urologists

G.W. Drach (✉)
Department of Surgery, Perelman Center for Advanced Medicine,
Hospital of the University of Pennsylvania, Philadelphia, PA 19104, USA
e-mail: drachg@uphs.upenn.edu

T.J. Guzzo et al. (eds.), *Primer of Geriatric Urology*, DOI 10.1007/978-1-4614-4773-3_1,   1
© Springer Science+Business Media New York 2013

Table 1.1 Outpatient visits, selected specialties, 2006. Percent outpatient Medicare clients

Specialty	Percent
Cardiovascular	58.4
Ophthalmology	48.5
Urology	47.9
Gen'l Int'l Med	42.7
Gen'l Surgery	35.8
Neurology	28.6
Dermatology	28.1
Family Practice	25.9
Orthopedic	25
Otolaryngology	22.5
Psychiatry	9.9
OB/GYN	7.1

Data selected from National Ambulatory Medical Care Survey, 2006

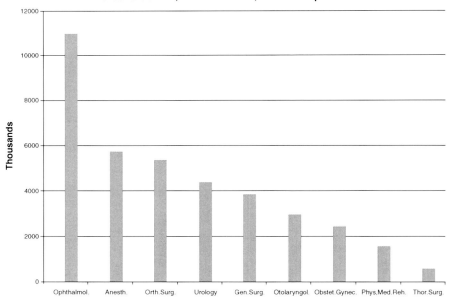

Persons Served, Medicare 2009, Selected Specialties

Fig. 1.1 Number of persons served by selected surgical and related specialties in the year 2009

and other surgical specialties increases for patients over age 65 (Fig. 1.2). And as of 2005–2006, prostate cancer became the eighth most common diagnosis for Medicare patients (Table 1.2).

Your elderly urologic patients merit special assessment on several fronts. Many nonoperative urologic conditions, such as lower urinary tract symptoms, require treatment with medications that can affect cognition and/or interact with other daily

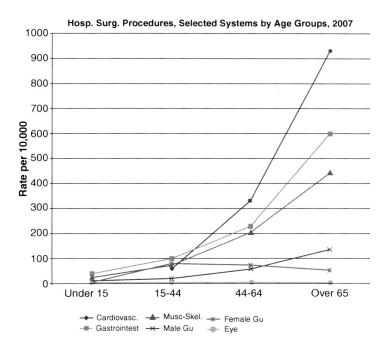

Fig. 1.2 In-hospital surgical procedures in rate per 10,000 persons, for selected surgical specialties. Note that urology and ophthalmology appear to have low rates. However, many of their procedures are performed in office or ambulatory facilities

Table 1.2 Most Common eight geriatric/Medicare diagnoses

Diagnosis	Percent, age 65+
Hypertension	53
Arthritis	49.6
Heart disease	31
Diabetes	18.1
Sinusitis	13.8
Ulcer	10.8
Asthma	10.6
Prostate cancer	10.2

Data from CDC trends in Health and Aging, 2005–2006

medications [1]. Urinary afflictions such as frequency, urgency, and incontinence contribute to non-urologic morbidity because of requirement for movement and result in falls. The need to arise at night for voiding (nocturia) also leads to increased risk of falls in the darkened environment. Older patients' needs differ because processes of aging make them different from those younger than 65 years. Why? Because the physiology of aging generates changes that cause the elderly to have

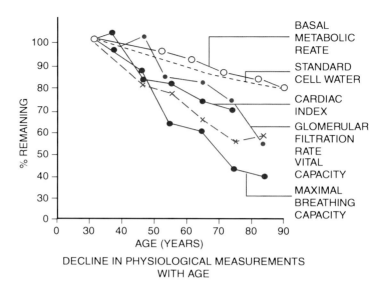

Fig. 1.3 Graphic depiction of deterioration of various body systems as one ages

less physiological strength in many organ systems. Perhaps one of the best illustrations of these changes is summarized in Fig. 1.3 [2]. Note that renal function decreases to 60% of normal by age 80, cardiac function by 30% and pulmonary function by 50–60%. Some geriatricians term this loss of reserve function in body systems as "homeostenosis" or lack of ability to respond adequately to external stresses, versus the usual beneficial response of "homeostasis"[3]. It is this inability to respond to stress that causes the increased risk levels that one tries to include in various co-morbidity classifications. And in addition to consideration of the usual disease conditions that one considers dangerous (hypertension, cardiovascular disease, pulmonary disease, diabetes, etc), there are a number of additional topics that pertain to the aged patient, termed "geriatric syndromes" (Table 1.3) [4].

Yet many patients over age 75 or 80 retain excellent physiologic function through a combination of physical conditioning and lack of chronic disease. Hence, it becomes critical to evaluate the older patient on a basis of *physiologic rather than chronologic* age. Several methods to predict likelihood of survival in years (remaining life span) or of operative risk exist. These include the Charlson Index (Table 1.4) and the Anesthesia Society of America (ASA) classification (Table 1.5) [5]. Use of these concepts of co-morbidity is brought together in the South Florida Treatment Algorithm (Table 1.6) [6]. In general, for patients with no co-morbidities, one estimates years of life remaining by using predictive graphs (Fig. 1.4). As illustrated, due to improvements in general health and medical care, the 2007 median life expectancy for an individual reaching age 65 was 17.1 years and at age 75 reached 10.7 years. And if the age achieved is 85, there is still an expectancy of 7 years.

Table 1.3 Geriatric syndromes

Deconditioning
Delirium
Dementia
Elder abuse
Falls
Frailty
Malnutrition
Osteoporosis
Palliative care/end of life
Polypharmacy
Pressure ulcers
Transitional Care
Urinary incontinence

Data from JAMA and Archives [4]

Table 1.4 Charlson score: weighted index of co-morbidity

Assigned weights for diseases conditions
1. Myocardial infarct
   Congestive heart failure
   Peripheral vascular disease
   Cerebrovascular disease
   Dementia
   Chronic pulmonary disease
   Connective tissue disease
   Ulcer disease
   Mild liver disease
   Diabetes
2. Hemiplegia
   Moderate or severe renal disease
   Diabetes with end organ damage
   Any tumor
   Leukemia
   Lymphoma
3. Moderate or severe liver disease
4. Metastatic solid tumor
   AIDS

Assigned weights for each condition that a patient has. The total equals the Charlson score. Example: chronic pulmonary (1) and lymphoma (2) = total score (3)

Urologists will be faced with the inevitable results of this growth of the elderly population, because we care for many elderly in our outpatient and inpatient practices. And, if you are like me, you had little or no previous education in the specifics of care of our older patients while in medical school or residency. Perhaps you could say that you did learn such things because you've had "on the job training," but

Table 1.5 American Society of Anesthesiologists physical status classification system

ASA physical status 1—A normal healthy patient

ASA physical status 2—A patient with mild systemic disease

ASA physical status 3—A patient with severe systemic disease

ASA physical status 4—A patient with severe systemic disease that is a constant threat to life

ASA physical status 5—A moribund patient who is not expected to survive without the operation

ASA physical status 6—A declared brain-dead patient whose organs are being removed for donor purposes

Data from American Society of Anesthesiologists [5]

Table 1.6 Concepts of adaption in treatment for the elderly

Basic principle: will you extend useful life if you treat/operate on this patient?

Impact of co-morbidities on life expectancy of elderly patient:

　　1.　Healthy at age 65 = expectancy 17 years, at 85 = expectancy 7 years

Offer normal treatment regimen

　　2.　Two or fewer co-morbidities = life expectancy less

Offer regimen adapted to co-morbidities

　　3.　More than two co-morbidities = expectancy much less

Treat to provide comfort and/or palliation

Adapted from Lichtman [6]

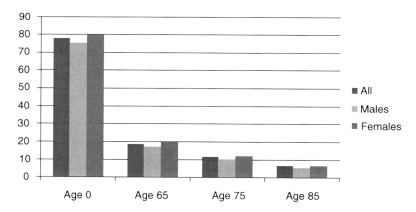

Fig. 1.4 Estimation of mean remaining lifetimes for individuals at birth and at ages 65, 75, and 85 for the year 2010

indeed that is not adequate for geriatrics just as it is not adequate for pediatrics. Many elderly urologic patients merit special assessment on several fronts. As noted above, many nonoperative urologic conditions (such as lower urinary tract symptoms) require medications that can affect cognition or interact with other daily medications. Which are these? Urinary incontinence or urgency and frequency can lead to related morbidities such as falls or loss of necessary sleep. Have these points already been considered? When surgical intervention is contemplated, critical elements such as degree of normal cognition, level of frailty, living conditions and sites of postsurgical aftercare must be considered. Do you know that nearly 1/3 of older women live by themselves and by age 85, 85% live alone [7]! Who takes care of them after surgical intervention?

Having, I believe, proved to you that most adult urologists have a significant geriatric practice, the next goal is to present to you the basics of effective evaluation and to prepare for effective management of the geriatric patient. Our next chapter will introduce you to the major additional points needed in the evaluation of the older patient. Thereafter you will be introduced to the major approaches you may take toward the elderly patient in your office procedures. Subsequent chapters will discuss medical therapy and procedural therapy. Then will follow a consideration of those complications peculiar to the older patient. Next, you will be exposed to use of adjunctive services and, possible, nursing home adjuncts. Finally, there will be coverage of those specific entities of geriatric urology: cancer, lower urinary tract symptoms, and sexuality.

Our purpose is to improve your care of the geriatric patient, to lubricate and ease your office procedures in the management of these patients and to promote effective decision making during hospitalization and treatment of the elderly patient, especially those considered to be the frail elderly. This will not be a comprehensive text, but as the title says, a "Primer" to help you gain additional fundamental knowledge that is important in the care of your geriatric patient.

References

1. Reuben DB, Herr KA, Pacala JT, et al. Geriatrics at your fingertips. New York: American Geriatrics Society; 2009.
2. Barnett S. Portal of Geriatric Online Education. 2011. Available from: http://www.pogoe.org/productid/18801. Accessed 27 June 2011.
3. Troncale JA. The aging process. Physiologic changes and pharmacologic implications. Postgrad Med. 1996;99:111–4.
4. JAMA and Archives. Continuing medical education. Available from: http://cmejama-archives.ama-assn.org/cgi/hierarchy/amacme_node;jama_topic_1.
5. American Society of Anesthesologists Physical Status Classification System. 2011. Available from: http://www.asahq.org/clinical/physicalstatus.htm. Accessed 27 June 2011.
6. Lichtman SM. Guidelines for the treatment of elderly patients. Cancer Control. 2003;10:445–53.
7. Crescioni M, Gorina Y, Bilheimer L, Gillum RF. 2010. Trends in health status and health care use among older men. National health statistics reports; no. 24. Hyattsville, MD: National Center for Health Statistics.

Chapter 2
Approach to the Elderly Patient: Evaluation

George W. Drach

Geriatric Urology adds a number of specific requirements to your knowledge and skill set in the evaluation and management of the elderly patient. One list summarizes a number of geriatric syndromes [1] that were unique to care of the elderly patient (Table 2.1). Including these domains into your original evaluation takes very little extra time, but it does take some extra attention. Throughout this Chapter, we will be referring to a small text published by the American Geriatrics Society entitled "Geriatrics at Your Fingertips [2]" (GAYF). It is available online or in print at http://geriatricsatyourfingertips.org/ and it is a recommended addition to your office library for your care of geriatric patients.

Several steps must be added to the usual initial history and physical assessment of your geriatric patient that will improve your ability to care for them as you proceed to your management phase. Your first additional step will be to determine the patient's *communication status*. Is there evidence or history of decreased hearing or vision? About 60% of older patients have difficulty with one or the other or both senses [3]. What is their medical literacy level? Again, at least 1/4 of patients have a lack of education or basic lack of understanding of common medical terms [4]. And with the growing number of legal or illegal immigrants into the USA, urologists are likely to see many persons from foreign countries with their own specific cultural prejudices regarding medical care. Often, a family member acts as the interpreter—but the patient may not wish to divulge all of their history through that person. Accordingly, your initial record should simply record at the outset these three points: adequacy of senses, medical literacy, and cultural background. Thereafter, if you proceed with various treatment plans you can account for these special needs, e.g., being sure to have hearing aids available in the ICU after surgery.

G.W. Drach (✉)
Department of Surgery, Perelman Center for Advanced Medicine,
Hospital of the University of Pennsylvania, Philadelphia, PA 19104, USA
e-mail: drachg@uphs.upenn.edu

T.J. Guzzo et al. (eds.), *Primer of Geriatric Urology*, DOI 10.1007/978-1-4614-4773-3_2,
© Springer Science+Business Media New York 2013

Table 2.1 Special syndromes of geriatric care [1]

Deconditioning
Delirium
Dementia
Falls
Frailty
Malnutrition
Osteoporosis
Palliative/end of life care
Polypharmacy
Pressure ulcers
Transitional care
Urinary incontinence

During acquisition of the history, some special inquiries must be added. One of the most important regards questions about present *prescription medications* as well as *all over-the-counter (OTC) drugs* including supplements, vitamins, and herbal/alternative therapies. Many elderly patients use such medications. For example, ingestion of significant amounts of ginseng can lead to bleeding complications [5, 6] (Lesson 33, Penn Chapter). Most older persons take multiple prescription medications. This will be discussed further in Chap. 4.

Additional questions must include the *functional capacity* of the individual. Can they still stoop, lift, reach, grasp, and walk adequately? About 28% of Medicare patients express some difficulty with these activities [3]. After you have undergone major abdominal surgery, grip strength status may not be recovered even 6 months after surgery in many patients [7]. If these functional abilities are limited before surgery, they will likely never be recovered, and your patient will require help to get the jar off the upper shelf and then open it. Also, many Medicare patients express difficulty with one or more of the ADL [8] (ADL) such as toileting, bathing, eating, dressing, grooming, or (as noted above) walking (Fig. 2.1). A quick ADL assessment will define where help may be needed. If and when discharge plans are to be made, the number of ADL disabilities will help determine the discharge site (See Chap. 7). And finally, one must assess and record the Instrumental Activities of Daily Living [9] (IADL), so named because they require some type of tool or instrument to accomplish them. They are phoning, shopping, cooking, cleaning, laundering, and traveling (Fig. 2.2). For example, can the patient phone the dispatcher to order a cab to go shopping for food and soap? Noting these points may seem onerous, but recording them during your initial encounter will save much time later in your course of care for the patient.

Estimating and maintaining functional status for your patient becomes one of the most critical portions of your geriatric care. In the past, Forciea and I [5] have indicated that "No element of the preoperative examination of the older patient is more predictive of perioperative morbidity and mortality than functional ability." If, for example, you doubt the patient's ability to "get about," you can easily include a brief "Get-Up-and-Go" test [10] into your office activities (Table 2.2). This might take

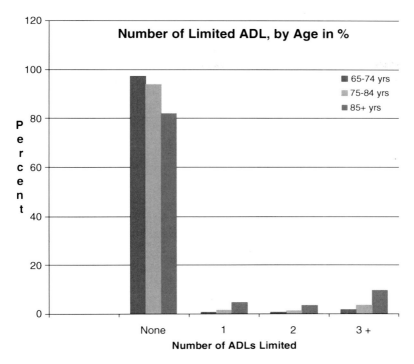

Fig. 2.1 Number of limited activities of daily living by age

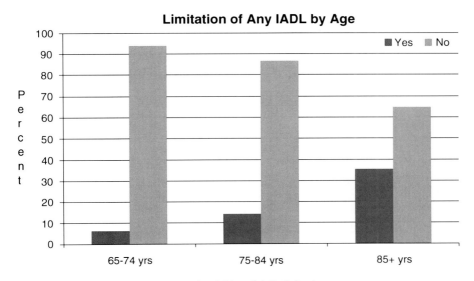

Fig. 2.2 Limitation of any instrumental activities of daily living by age

Table 2.2 Get-up-and-go test

Patient sitting in chair
Stand without using arms for boost or support
Walk 10 ft, turn around and return to chair
Sit without using arms for support
Some prefer to time test: if time <15 s test is good [11]

Observations: Are there any unusual movements? Balanced? No weaving or hesitancy? Regular steps without difficulty? If no problems, mobility function should be adequate

Table 2.3 Mini-mental status evaluation (GAYF)

1. With patient's attention, mention three unrelated words that are to be remembered
2. Ask the patient to draw a clock face with a specific time, such as 8:20
3. Then have the patient repeat the three words in 1. Above

Grading: Give one point for each word remembered. Give 2 points for a normal clock face. 0–2 points suspicious for dementia

one of your office staff 2–3 min, but doing so will save you many hours if your patient cannot ambulate after surgery [11, 12].

As you go through these prior points in acquiring the history, you will be making observations about the patient's *mental status and likely competency*. At some point you may begin to question the patient's mental state or the companion/caregiver may mention concern about the patient's mental ability. Two simple helps can be applied. First, the Mini-Mental Status examination can be done [13] (again by your trained office staff) (Table 2.3). It is available in GAYF also. If this suggests problems, you may want to request additional geriatric and/or psychiatric examinations. Second, it you question the patient's understanding of your descriptions of their problem or of your treatment plan, it is helpful to use the "repeat back" system. This requires that the patient "repeat back" to you so that *you* can understand what you have offered [14]. If you judge that the "repeat back" is adequate, it is useful to enter into the record your written confirming note. Then the patient and possible companion can sign along with you (this is still possible during these days of electronic records). If the above two processes create for you continued concern in the absence of a spouse or guardian, then it is advisable to determine whether someone is or could be created as a guardian for your patient. *Every county* in the USA has an office on aging that your patient's family or companion can contact for advice on this subject. Their office names may be unusual. As an example, for Philadelphia, the office is titled the "Philadelphia Corporation for Aging," but services for the elderly are available.

About 1/3 of all elderly patients who present with an urgent or emergent problem will manifest some *degree of malnutrition* [15]. As we all know, these patients heal poorly, have poor immune response, and encounter many more postoperative complications. Some initial hints may appear: weight loss of >10 lb in the past 6 months, body-mass-index (BMI) of under 22 or serum albumen of less than 3.0 on multi-test chemical panel (GAYF). Treatments by means of intravenous alimentation and so forth may result in some improvement [16]. If time allows, the production of improved nutrition in conjunction with a trained dietician provides the best resolution. However, if intervention is urgent, one must caution the family/friends that the risk is much higher for that patient. Under-nutrition, for example, clearly enhances the likelihood of pressure ulcers [17].

As mentioned above, many elderly single women in the USA or Great Britain live alone [18]. What is your *patient's living and social environment*? Who will care for them after their procedure? Do they have easy access to a kitchen or toilet and a bedroom on a single floor or are many steps up or down required? So knowledge of living arrangements and social status become important in your initial records, especially if you are to progress to some major procedural/operative intervention. Here again, if you have significant questions about the home situation, you might obtain assistance from a nearby social service group, often found in your local hospital or in conjunction with the county aging office, mentioned above.

Although frequently mentioned in popular literature, it is surprising how many elderly patients have not initiated their Living Will or Health Care Power of Attorney (HCPOA) or Physicians Orders for Life Sustaining Treatment (POLST) (GAYF). Availability of such *legal documents* should be noted, and if not done, your patient should be encouraged to accomplish this before even the simplest of procedures.

So now we have covered most of the additional historical knowledge that you must obtain in order to do your best for your geriatric urology patient. These points are summarized in Table 2.4 as a quick reminder. Cudennec et al. [19] have called completion of these steps a "Simplified Geriatric Assessment," and they found it to be an "important aid to decision making in the management of elderly patients with bronchial cancer." It seems that it can be just as useful in urology.

We will assume that your usual general questions and specific urologic system inquiries for voiding difficulty, sexual function, presence or absence of incontinence, histories of urologic diseases such as infection, calculi, or carcinoma have been completed.

Next, one performs the appropriate physical examination for the patient. This may be a head-to-toe complete physical examination or a system limited physical, depending on your analysis of the chief complaint. In addition to your usual observations, some general conditions may be noted and important in your future care of the patient. These include evidence of frailty, or "a transitional state in the dynamic progression from robustness to functional decline." It is further characterized by the fact that no single system is altered, but multiple systems are involved [20, 21].

However, performance of the above thorough history and examination will uncover the clues necessary to diagnose frailty: appearance not consistent with age, poor nutrition, poor subjective health rating, poor mental and physical performance, decreased sensory status and inadequate current living and care levels. Frail patients demonstrate a much higher risk of morbidity and mortality after any intervention. Other geriatric syndromes that may be noted on your examination (Table 2.1) are osteoporosis, arthritis, or limited mobility. These may strongly impact your ability to position the patient for various procedures. An inquiry about falls within the past year may provide a hint about difficulty in ambulation and balance and enable you to initiate special protections if the patient is to be hospitalized.

Table 2.4 Considerations in the initial evaluation of the geriatric patient

Communication status:
Decreased hearing or vision?
Medical literacy level
Cultural or language barriers
Prescription medications, OTC drugs, supplements, and alternative therapies
Functional status:
Physical capacities: stooping, lifting, reaching, grasping, and walking
Activities of Daily Living (ADL): toilet, bathe, eat, dress, groom, walk
Instrumental Activities of Daily Living (IADL): phone, shop, cook, tidy up, launder, travel
Cognitive status and competency
Nutritional status
Living arrangements and social status
Legal documents

Table 2.5 Indications for preoperative testing (adapted from Hepner [22])

Diagnostic efficacy: does the test correctly identify abnormalities?
Diagnostic effectiveness: would the test change your diagnosis?
Therapeutic efficacy: would the test change your management?
Therapeutic effectiveness: would the test change the patient's outcome?

Table 2.6 Preoperative consultation recommended for patients with these conditions

Recent myocardial disease/angina
Arrythmias
Aortic stenosis
Chronic lung disease
Renal or hepatic failure
Diabetes mellitus
Dementia or history of delirium

Of course, once you have covered these points in your history and physical examination, you will be looking for additional laboratory tests that might help you beyond the usual CBC and urinalysis. Some no longer recommend "routine" preoperative laboratory testing, but indicate that your requests should be based on your expectations of need [22], as illustrated in Table 2.5. Then, if your suspicions of potential difficulty increase after the initial history, physical examination and preliminary laboratory tests, you may feel the need for additional consultation. Table 2.6 depicts those conditions that should be evaluated by a specialist in that area (GAYF). But other suspicions should engender other consultations. Or perhaps a "Comprehensive Geriatric Assessment" may be in order, if you have a geriatrician nearby [23]. However, if, at this point you feel that you find your patient healthy and with minimal morbidity for his or her age, you may feel confident that you have performed your evaluation with the necessary added geriatric components and proceed with some degree of confidence. In our next chapter, you will be reminded of approaches to the specifics of urologic office procedures in the elderly patient.

References

1. Arizona Health Sciences Library. Aging-related topics. 2011. Available from: http://www.ahsl.arizona.edu/topics/geriatrics. Accessed 18 Feb 2011.
2. Reuben DB, Herr HA, Pacala JT, et al. Geriatrics at your fingertips. New York: The American Geriatrics Society; 2009.
3. Campbell VA, Crews JE, Moriarty DG, et al. Surveillance for sensory impairment, activity limitation and health-related quality of life among older adults—United States, 1993–1997. MMWR. 1999;48:131–57.
4. Teutsch C. Patient-doctor communications. Med Clin North Am. 2003;87:1115–45.
5. Drach GW, Forciea MA. American Urological Association Update Series. American Urological Association 2005;24:287–95.
6. Drach GW. Geriatric urology. In: Hanno PJ, Malkowicz SB, Wein AJ, editors. Penn Clinical Manual of Urology. Philadelphia: WB Saunders; 2007.
7. Mathur S, Plank LD, Hill AG, et al. Changes in body composition, muscle function and energy expenditure after radical cystectomy. BJU Int. 2007;101:973–7.
8. Centers for Disease Control and Prevention. Limitations in activities of daily living and instrumental activities of daily living, 2003–2007. 2011. Available from: http://www.cdc.gov/nchs/health_policy/ADL_tables.htm. Accessed 29 June 2011.
9. Centers for Disease Control and Prevention. Instrumental activities of daily living. 2011. Available from: http://www.cdc.gov/nchs/health_policy/IADL_tables.htm. Accessed 29 June 2011.
10. Gericareonline.net. Get-up-and-go test. Available from: http://gericareonline.net/tools/eng/falls/attachments/Falls_Tool_2_Get_Up_and_GoTest.pdf.
11. Nordin E, Lindelof N, Rosendahl E, et al. Prognostic validity of the Timed Up-and-Go test, a modified Get-up-and-Go test, staff's global judgment and fall history in evaluating fall risk in residential fare facilities. Age Ageing. 2008;37:442–8.
12. Malani PS. Functional status assessment in the preoperative evaluation of older adults. JAMA. 2009;302:1582–3.
13. Gericareonline.net. Mini mental status exam. Available from: http://gericareonline.net/tools/eng/attachments/ML_Tool2_Brief_Screening_Tools.pdf
14. Fink AS, Prochazka AV, Henderson WG, et al. Enhancement of surgical informed consent by addition of repeat back: a multicenter, randomized controlled clinical trial. Ann Surg. 2010;252:27–36.
15. Ahmed T, Haboubi N. Assessment and management of nutrition in older people and its importance to health. Clin Interv Aging. 2010;5:207–16.
16. Botella-Carretero JI, Iglesias B, Balsa JA, et al. Perioperative oral nutrition supplements in normally or mildly undernourished geriatric patients submitted to surgery for hip fracture: a randomized clinical trial. Clin Nutr. 2011;29:574–9.
17. Botella-Carretero JI, Balsa JA. Perioperative oral nutrition supplements in normally or mildly undernourished geriatric patients submitted to surgery for hip fracture: a randomized clinical trial: response to letter to the editor. Clin Nutr. 2011;30:398.
18. UK National Statistics. 2011. Available from: http://www.statistics.gov.uk. Accessed 27 June 2011.
19. Cudennec T, Gendry T, Labrune S, et al. Use of a simplified geriatric evaluation in thoracic oncology. Lung Cancer. 2010;67:232–6.
20. Lang P, Michel J, Zekry D. Frailty syndrome: a transitional state in a dynamic process. Gerontology. 2009;55:539–49.
21. Makary MA, Degev DL, Pronovost PJ, et al. Frailty as a predictor of surgical outcomes in older patients. J Am Coll Surg. 2010;210:901–8.
22. Hepner DI. The role of testing in the preoperative evaluation. Cleve Clin J Med. 2009;76:822–7.
23. Kristjansson SR, Nesbakken A, Jordhey MS, et al. Comprehensive geriatric assessment can predict complications in elderly patients after elective surgery for colorectal cancer: a prospective observational cohort study. Crit Rev Oncol Hematol. 2010;76:208–17.

Chapter 3
Urologic Office Procedures

Sanjay Kasturi, William I. Jaffe, and Ariana L. Smith

Introduction

Office procedures are an important part of any urologic practice. Given the prevalence of urologic disease in the elderly population, it is paramount to understand the special considerations when performing office procedures in this population. This section will review common urologic office procedures with emphasis on care of the geriatric patient.

Positioning for Office Procedures

Simple procedures such as catheterizations and flexible cystoscopy may be performed in the supine position in men and in the "frog-legged" position in women. More complex office procedures requiring rigid cystoscopy will require the patient to be placed in the lithotomy position. In the lithotomy position the patient is supine with their buttocks at the end of the exam table, the legs are placed in stirrups such that the angle of flexion at the hips and knees are no more than 90°, and the hips are abducted generally no more than 30°. Examples of the "standard" and "low" lithotomy

S. Kasturi (✉)
Resident in Urology, Hospital of the University of Pennsylvania,
Philadelphia, PA 19104, USA
e-mail: sanjay.kasturi@uphs.upenn.edu

W.I. Jaffe
Department of Surgery, Division of Urology, Penn Presbyterian Hospital,
Philadelphia, PA 19104, USA

A.L. Smith
Department of Urology, Hospital of the University of Pennsylvania and Pennsylvania Hospital,
Philadelphia, PA 19106, USA

T.J. Guzzo et al. (eds.), *Primer of Geriatric Urology*, DOI 10.1007/978-1-4614-4773-3_3,
© Springer Science+Business Media New York 2013

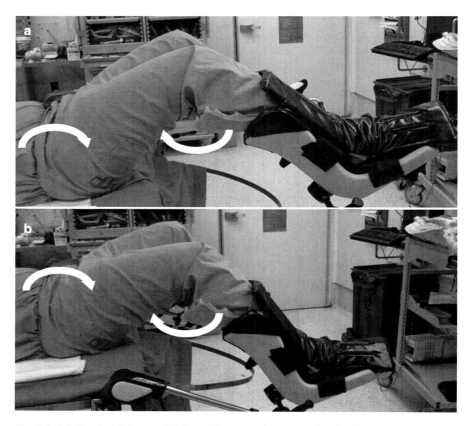

Fig. 3.1 (**a**) Standard lithotomy (**b**) Low lithotomy, please note that the hip and knee joints are flexed no more than 90° and pressure points are padded (foam)

position are shown in Fig. 3.1. The prevalence of joint disorders and prosthetics and in the elderly patient needs to be taken into account. For instance, it is estimated that per age group patients aged >65 years are 3.5–4.5 times more likely to undergo total hip arthroplasty than patients <65 years [1]. Foam or gel padding of the ankles, calves, and knees are advocated to release pressure on these areas. This position is generally well tolerated in the office; complications such as compartment syndrome tend to occur in the operating room when surgical times exceed 4–6 h [2].

Catheterization

Catheterization may be needed in several scenarios in the office setting. Non-indwelling or straight catheterization may be used to obtain a sterile specimen for urine culture or, to determine post-void residual (PVR) urine volume. An indwelling catheter is generally placed due to urinary retention. The insertion and maintenance of catheters are important for the elderly population and their caregivers, since roughly 5–10% of all nursing home patients and up to 18% of nursing home patient with lower urinary tract symptoms (LUTS) have Foley catheters [3, 4]. General catheter care involves maintaining a closed drainage system to avoid ascending infection, regularly cleaning of the area that exits the genitalia to prevent encrustation and irritation, and most importantly, removal of the indwelling catheter at the earliest possible time point. Long-term indwelling catheterization is not ideal management due to recurrent infections, urethral erosion, and loss of cyclical bladder function. In patients who are unable to void spontaneously, self-intermittent catheterization is preferred with suprapubic tube drainage (see below) as an alternative option for those patients who are unable to perform self-intermittent catheterization.

Sterile technique including sterile gloves, cleansing of the urethra and surrounding genitalia, and use of a sterile catheter is recommended in the office or hospital setting. Self-intermittent catheterization does not require sterile technique, but hand washing and avoidance of gross contamination is recommended. Liberal use of lubricating jelly or 2% lidocaine jelly will aid the ease in passage of the catheter. At times difficulty is encountered when passing a catheter due to an enlarged prostate, a false passage, a bladder neck contracture, or a urethral stricture. In these scenarios a coude catheter, a guide wire with council tip catheter, or filiforms and followers may be needed (Fig. 3.2).

Urethral Dilation

In the setting of urethral stricture or meatal stenosis urethral dilation may be necessary. A local anesthetic is administered prior to instrumentation. It is critical that the lumen of the stricture be intubated properly to avoid creation of a false passage. The safest method is to use a cystoscope and pass a wire through the narrowed lumen under direct visualization. Over the wire sequential dilators are generally passed until an appropriate luminal diameter is achieved (Fig. 3.3). Urethral sound may be more appropriate in the rare but often over-diagnosed female urethral stricture (Fig. 3.3). Following dilation the physician may place a temporary indwelling catheter to keep the area open, recommended intermittent self-catheterization, or simply have the patient return to the office at a designated time point for interval evaluation.

Cystoscopy

Cystoscopy or cystourethroscopy, is a procedure that allows visualization of the entire bladder and urethra. This can be performed in the office under local anesthesia (2% lidocaine jelly or intravesicle lidocaine). The cystoscope can be flexible or rigid depending on the needs of the patient or the positioning of the patient (Fig. 3.4).

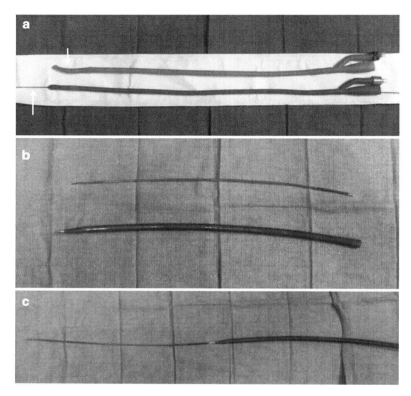

Fig. 3.2 (a) Coude catheter on *top*, *arrow* highlights curved tip that allows this catheter to pass through an enlarged prostate, council catheter on *bottom*, *arrow* highlights ability of this catheter to be passed over a wire (b) Filiform on *top*, this instrument in soft and pliable that allows it to traverse a stricture, follower on *bottom*, this instrument is the dilating element (c) Filiform and follower connected

Flexible cystoscopy may be performed supine, but rigid cystoscopy requires the lithotomy position. For the comfort of the patient, the smallest diameter cystoscope should be used during rigid cystoscopy (17 French). To aid in visualization a sterile fluid, generally normal saline, is used to distend the urethra and bladder. Biopsies can be obtained by passing forceps through the working channel of the cystoscope. Fulguration of biopsy sites or other areas of the bladder can be performed using Bugbee electrocautery, however glycine, sorbitol, or water must be used as the irrigant. Laser ablation of bladder tumors, lesions, or stones can be performed using various wavelengths of laser energy and specific laser fibers.

Reasonable effort should be made to ensure that the patient has sterile urine before proceeding with any urological instrumentation. Current evidence suggests that in uncomplicated situations antibiotics are not required or recommended. In patients with total joint replacements, prophylaxis is recommended in those who have been implanted within the last 2 years and those patients who are high risk

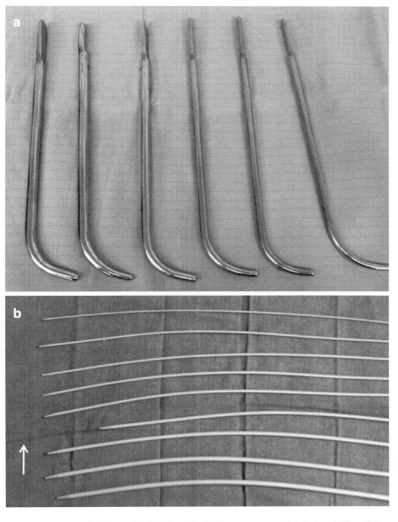

Fig. 3.3 (**a**) Serial sound dilators (**b**) Serial urethral dilators, *arrow* highlights ability of these dilator to be passed over a wire

(inflammatory arthropathies, immunosuppressed, previous joint infections) [5]. Prophylaxis is not needed in patients with plates, pins, or screws. Currently, the American Heart Association (AHA) does not recommend antibiotic prophylaxis for patients with undergoing urologic procedures for the prevention of infectious endocarditis [6]. Discontinuation of blood thinning agent is not needed in all situations but the physician should be made aware of any blood thinning medications (aspirin, ibuprofen, warfarin, antiplatelet agents). If additional treatment through the cystoscope is anticipated blood thinners should be stopped. Lastly, several authors have

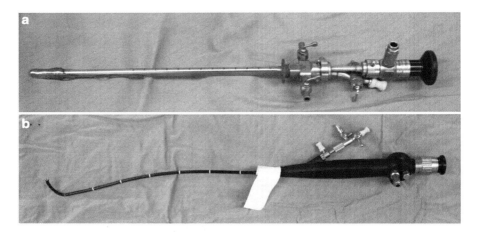

Fig. 3.4 (a) Rigid cystoscope (b) Flexible cystoscopy

noted that bactrim and fluoroquinolones can lead to supratherapeutic INR levels in patients taking coumadin [7]. If these antibiotics are given after cystoscopy, appropriate communication with primary care doctors and geriatric practitioners is needed for INR monitoring in elderly patients taking coumadin.

Side effects of cystoscopy are generally mild. They may include dysuria, hematuria, difficulty urinating, and rarely urinary tract infection. Complications are rare but may include stricture formation, acute urinary retention, bleeding, and clot retention.

Suprapubic Tube Placement

Suprapubic tubes (SPTs) are often employed in urology for patients with neurogenic bladder (who cannot perform intermittent straight catheterization) or when urethral access to the bladder is not feasible (trauma, severe stricture disease). Two recent large studies of 219 and 549 patients each, found that the average age at time of SPT placement was 73 years and 66 years of age, respectively [8, 9]. As such, it is important that elderly patients, their families, and primary caregivers be aware of long-term common complications of SPTs such as urinary tract infections and catheter blockages.

Placement of a suprapubic tube is best performed in the operating room in a controlled setting either through an open incision or percutaneously (with or without the aid of cystoscopy and/or ultrasound). Placement of an SPT in the office should be reserved for emergency situations and should be aided by cystoscopy if feasible as serious complications such as bowel injury, vascular injury, and SPT misplacement can occur.

When performed in the office, the bladder should first be fully distended. Then after local anesthesia is given, a small transverse skin incision should be made about

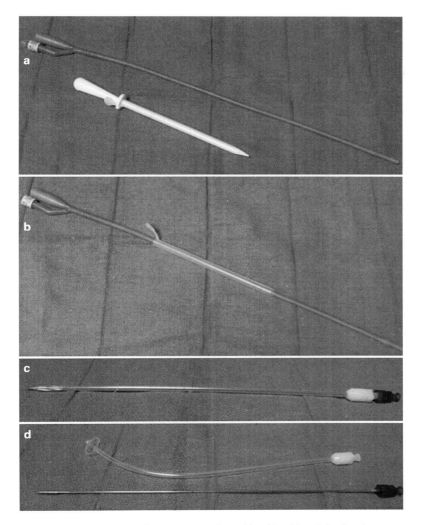

Fig. 3.5 (**a, b**) Rousch trocar (**c, d**) cystotomy catheter kit with self retaining head

3–4 cm (or two finger-breaths) above the pubis. Next, a long spinal or "finder" needle should be placed perpendicular to the skin and not too cephalad (away from the bladder) or too caudad (too close to the bladder neck). Urine should be aspirated from the spinal needle to confirm placement if a cystoscopy is not already in the bladder to confirm placement. Next, either a Rousch trocar or cystotomy catheter kit may be inserted in the same direction and aside the spinal needle. For the Rousch trocar, a catheter is placed through the hollow lumen, which is then "peeled" away (Fig. 3.5). For the cystotomy catheter kit, the obturator is removed leaving the catheter in place (Fig. 3.5).

SPT care is similar to an indwelling urethral catheter (see above). Most urologist exchange SPTs every month in the office, however if encrustation and occlusion are a problem, then exchange may be needed every 2–3 weeks.

Urodynamics

Urodynamics is an important aspect of any urologic practice. Elderly patients may be referred for urodynamics for a variety of reason including bladder outlet obstruction, pelvic organ prolapse, overactive bladder, and urinary incontinence. Of all these reasons, urinary incontinence is perhaps the most bothersome to elderly patients and their caregivers. In fact, incontinence affects as many as 40% of patients in nursing homes and accounts for a significant amount of urodynamic referrals in this population. This sect. will define the urodynamic evaluation as standardized by the International Continence Society (ICS) [10], and will discuss when relevant specific application to the elderly population.

Noninvasive uroflowmetry is the simplest methodology in urodynamics. It should be noted that this method is largely dependent on voided volume (minimum of 150 cc required) and a normal maximum flow rate is derived from nomograms based on age and sex. In men, the lowest acceptable maximum flow rates are 21 mL/s, 12 mL/s, and 9 mL/s in age groups of 14–45 years, 46–65 years, and 66–80 years respectively. In women maximum flow rates are 18 mL/s, 15 mL/s, and 10 mL/s in age groups of 14–45 years, 46–65 years, and 66–80 years respectively [11]. In general, most people would accept >15 mL/s as normal [12]. Figure 3.6 [13] represents the ideal uroflowmetry curve and Table 3.1 defines the terminology [10]. In combination with uroflowmetry, post-void residual urine measurement (PVR) urine completes the noninvasive urodynamic evaluation. PVR measurements are typically assessed by ultrasound exam (or catheterization) within 60 s of voiding. Any further delay in PVR measurements risks a false elevation in the value from continued urine production. The definition of an elevated PVR is not standardized, but a value of greater than 50–100 cc is generally accepted as elevated depending on the clinical situation. Interestingly, PVR is not affected by age of male patients, however in randomly selected men aged 70–79 years about 25% will have a PVR greater than 50 mL [14].

Cystometry refers to the measurement of the pressure/volume relationship of the bladder during filling and voiding. Cystometrogram is the graphical recording of the bladder pressures and volume over time during the filling phase, which commences when filling starts and ends when the patient is given permission to void (Fig. 3.7) [13].

The goals of filling cystometry are to assess bladder sensation, bladder capacity, detrusor overactivity, and bladder compliance. Filling itself may be at a physiologic rate, which is less than the predicted maximum (i.e., body weight in kilograms divided by 4, expressed as mL/min) or non-physiologic (i.e., greater than the predicted maximum). Common filling rates used in practice are 10–100 mL per minute.

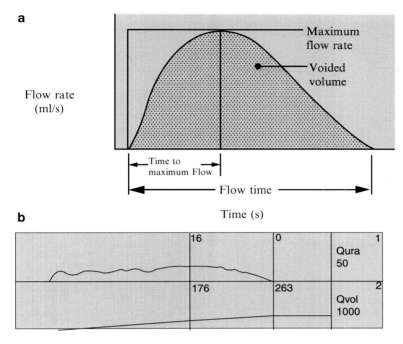

Fig. 3.6 (**a, b**) The ideal flow curve (from Peterson and Webster [13]; with permission from Saunders-Elsevier)

Table 3.1 Uroflowmetry

Term (units)	Definition
Urine flow	Voluntary urethral passage of urine described in terms of flow rate and flow pattern
	Flow pattern may be either continuous (no interruption) or Intermittent (interruptions present)
Flow rate (mL/s)	Volume of urine expelled via the urethra per unit time
Voided volume (mL)	Total amount of urine expelled via the urethra
Maximum urine flow rate (mL/s)-Qmax	Maximum measured value of the flow rate correcting for artifact
Flow time (sec)	The time over which measurable flow actually occurs
Average Urine flow rate (mL/s)-Qave	Voided volume divided by the flow time
Voiding time (s)	Duration of the void including interruptions, voiding time equals flow time when voiding is completed without interruptions
Time to maximum flow (s)	Elapsed time from the onset of urine flow to maximum urine flow

Bladder sensation is assessed by questioning the patient. These parameters are detailed in Table 3.2 [10]. Pain during filling is abnormal and should be noted by the clinician.

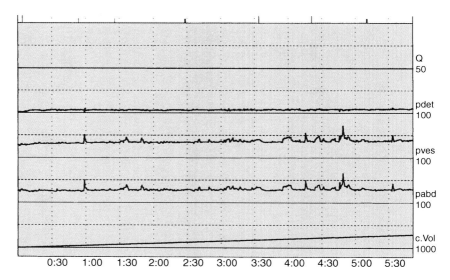

Fig. 3.7 Normal cystogram, please note normal compliance and no detrusor overactivity (from Peterson and Webster [13]; with permission from Saunders-Elsevier)

Bladder capacity may be assessed in several ways. The first is the functional bladder capacity, which is the largest volume voiding in a voiding diary [13]. Second, cystometric capacity is the bladder volume when the patient is given permission to void and maximum cystometric capacity is the bladder volume when the patient can no longer delay micturition [10].

Normal detrusor function during filling cystometry is defined as little or no change in detrusor pressure with filling. Furthermore, there are no involuntary phasic contractions despite provocative maneuvers (rapid filling, use of cooled or acidic medium, postural changes, and hand washing). Detrusor overactivity refers to the involuntary contractions during filling that may be spontaneous or provoked producing a waveform of variable duration and amplitude. Relevant terminology to detrusor overactivity is listed in Table 3.3 [10].

The final component of filling cystometry is compliance. Compliance is defined as the change in bladder volume divide by the change in detrusor pressure during the change in bladder volume and it is expressed as mL per cm H_2O. The ICS recommends two distinct points on the CMG to calculate compliance: (1) Starting point for compliance is the detrusor pressure at the start of bladder filling and the corresponding volume (usually zero); (2) End point for compliance is the detrusor pressure and bladder volume at cystometric capacity (or immediately before the start of any detrusor contraction that causes significant leakage). Abnormally low compliance (<12.5 mL/cm H_2O) is a risk factor for renal deterioration caused by elevated bladder storage pressures.

Lastly, leakage of urine during filling cystometry should also be assessed for and described in detail. Urodynamic stress incontinence (replaces genuine

Table 3.2 Clinical parameters for bladder sensation

Term	Definition
First sensation of bladder filling	Sensation when the patient first becomes aware of bladder filling
First desire to void	First feeling that the patient may wish to pass urine
Normal desire to void	The feeling that leads the patient to pass urine at the next convenient moment, but voiding can be delayed
Strong desire to void	The persistent desire to pass urine without the fear of leakage
Urgency	Sudden, compelling desire to pass urine which is difficult to defer
Bladder oversensitivity	Increased perceived bladder sensation during bladder filling with (1) an early first desire to void (2) an early strong desire to void, which occurs at low bladder volumes (3) low cystometric bladder capacity (4) no abnormal increase in detrusor pressure
Reduced bladder sensation	Bladder sensation is perceived to be diminished during filling cystometry
Absent bladder sensation	The patient reports no bladder sensation during filling cystometry

Table 3.3 Detrusor overactivity terminology

Term	Definition
Phasic detrusor overactivity	Characteristic wave form and may or may not lead to urinary incontinence
Terminal detrusor overactivity	Single, involuntary detrusor contraction occurring at cystometric capacity which cannot be suppressed and results in incontinence usually with bladder emptying
Idiopathic detrusor overactivity	When no defined cause for detrusor overactivity (replaces detrusor instability)
Neurogenic detrusor overactivity	When there is a relevant neurological condition in the setting of detrusor overactivity

stress incontinence) is the involuntary leakage of urine during filling cystometry, associated with increased intra-abdominal pressures, in the absence of a detrusor contraction.

Abdominal leak point pressure (ALPP) is a dynamic pressure induced by an increase in abdominal pressure (cough or valsalva) and is measured at the lowest value of increased intravesical pressure that provokes urinary leakage in the absence of a detrusor contraction. It is assessed at a fixed bladder volume (at least 150–200 mL) and is used as an objective measure of stress urinary incontinence in women [13]. Typically ALPP of less than 60 cm H_2O indicates intrinsic sphincter deficiency (ISD), a value of 60–90 cm H_2O suggests a combination of ISD and urethral hypermobility, and a value of greater 90 cm H_2O suggests primarily urethral hypermobility. Detrusor leak point pressure (DLPP) is a static pressure measured as the lowest value of the detrusor pressure at which leakage is observed in the absence of increased abdominal pressure or a detrusor contraction. This is generally seen in patients with poor bladder compliance. In these instances, urethral leakage is essentially a "pop-off" mechanism. McGuire first described DLPP in a pediatric population

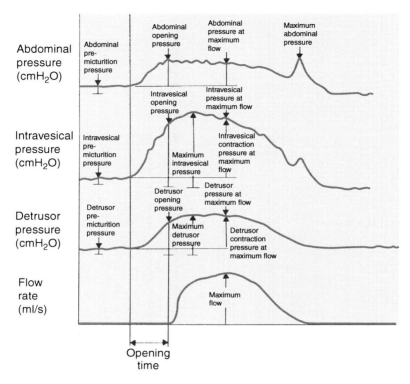

Fig. 3.8 Pressure flow study (from Peterson and Webster [13]; with permission from Saunders-Elsevier)

of patients with myelodysplasia [15]. In this setting, patients with DLPP greater than 40 cm of H_2O were at significant risk of upper tract deterioration than those with pressures less than 40 cm of H_2O. There are no data on a similar relationship in patients without neurological disease.

A pressure flow study is the graphical recording of the pressure volume relationship of the bladder during emptying, which beings when patient is given permission to void and ends when the patient considers their voiding has finished. A pressure flow study is depicted in Fig. 3.8 [13] and its terminology is described in Table 3.4 [10].

As defined by the ICS, normal voiding is achieved first by voluntary relaxation of the urinary sphincter (i.e., reduction in intra-urethral pressure) followed by a continuous detrusor contraction leading to complete bladder emptying within a normal time span [10]. Conversely, detursor underactivity (DU) is defined as a contraction of reduced strength and/or duration resulting in prolonged bladder emptying and/or a failure to achieve complete bladder emptying within a normal time span in the absence of obstruction.

Table 3.4 Pressure flow

Term	Definition
Premicturition pressure	Pressure recorded immediately before the initial isovolumetric contraction
Opening time	Time elapsed from initial rise in pressure to the onset of flow and reflects the time taken for fluid to pass from the point of pressure measurement to the uroflow transducer
Opening pressure	The pressure recorded at the onset of measured flow
Maximum pressure	Maximum value of the measured pressure
Pressure at maximum flow	Pressure recorded at the end of measured flow
Contraction pressure at maximum flow	Difference between the pressure at maximum flow and the premicturition pressure
Flow delay	Delay in time between a change in pressure and the corresponding change in measure flow rate

DU is a clinical syndrome that can be due to many causes such as fecal impaction, diabetes, medication, and impaired mobility [3]. It has been shown that detrusor function declines with age and is under-diagnosed in the geriatric population as a cause of LUTS. Impaired detrusor contractility (IDC) is used to describe this functional loss in detrusor strength. Interestingly, urodynamic studies in elderly institutionalized patients with urinary incontinence revealed that overall 61% suffer from uninhibited detrusor contractions and that half of these patients also have IDC [16]. This entity of DU with IDC and involuntary contractions is known as detrusor hyperactivity impaired contractility (DHIC). More recent data has shown that DU with IDC is present in 48% of elderly men and 12% of elderly women in the community presenting with LUTS. Furthermore, two thirds of these men and one half of these women had concomitant DHIC [4]. These results underscore the importance of recognizing DHIC during office urodynamics.

Lastly, video urodynamics utilizes fluoroscopy to visualize the lower urinary tract during filling cystometry and pressure flow urodynamics. It may be utilized when assessing for a specific site of obstruction (bladder neck dysfunction), unexplained retention in women, pelvic organ prolapse, neurogenic voiding dysfunction, and complex incontinence. Clearly many of these clinical situations are present in the elderly patient with LUTS.

Conclusions

This chapter set out to describe basic urologic office procedures and how these must be adapted to meet the needs of the elderly population. Specific attention must to be paid to patient positioning. Furthermore, urologic practitioners should be updated on indications for antibiotic prophylaxis as total joint replacements and valvular heart diseases are not uncommon in the elderly. Patients and caregivers must also be educated on proper care of indwelling catheters as these are often used to manage the lower urinary tract of the geriatric population. Finally, urologists must also be aware of changes in the lower urinary tract with age and be able to adjust for this when performing noninvasive urodynamics (uroflow and PVR) and be able to recognize DHIC on cystometry and pressure flow studies. This level of alertness to the urologic care of the elderly will ultimately benefit not only patients but also their caregivers and families.

Acknowledgment   The section on "Urodynamics" was adapted with permission from Kasturi S, Jaffe WI, Smith AL: Clinically relevant terminology of the lower female genitourinary tract. Curr Bladder Dysfunct Rep. 2011;6:159–166.

References

1. Kurtz S, Mowat F, Ong K, Chan N, Lau E, Halpern M. Prevalence of primary and revision total hip and knee arthroplasty in the United States from 1990 through 2002. J Bone Joint Surg Am. 2005;87(7):1487–97.
2. Raza A, Byrne D, Townell N. Lower limb (well leg) compartment syndrome after urological pelvic surgery. J Urol. 2004;171(1):5–11.
3. Taylor 3rd JA, Kuchel GA. Detrusor underactivity: clinical features and pathogenesis of an underdiagnosed geriatric condition. J Am Geriatr Soc. 2006;54(12):1920–32.
4. Abarbanel J, Marcus EL. Impaired detrusor contractility in community-dwelling elderly presenting with lower urinary tract symptoms. Urology. 2007;69(3):436–40.
5. American Urological Association; American Academy of Orthopaedic Surgeons. Antibiotic prophylaxis for urological patients with total joint replacements. J Urol. 2003;169:1796–7.
6. Wilson W, Taubert KA, Gewitz M, et al. Prevention of infective endocarditis: guidelines from the American Heart Association: a guideline from the American Heart Association Rheumatic Fever, Endocarditis and Kawasaki Disease Committee, Council on Cardiovascular Disease in the Young, and the Council on Clinical Cardiology, Council on Cardiovascular Surgery and Anesthesia, and the Quality of Care and Outcomes Research Interdisciplinary Working Group. J Am Dent Assoc. 2008;139(Suppl):3S–24.
7. Glasheen JJ, Fugit RV, Prochazka AV. The risk of overanticoagulation with antibiotic use in outpatients on stable warfarin regimens. J Gen Intern Med. 2005;20(7):653–6.
8. Cronin CG, Prakash P, Gervais DA, et al. Imaging-guided suprapubic bladder tube insertion: experience in the care of 549 patients. AJR Am J Roentgenol. 2011;196(1):182–8.
9. Ahluwalia RS, Johal N, Kouriefs C, Kooiman G, Montgomery BS, Plail RO. The surgical risk of suprapubic catheter insertion and long-term sequelae. Ann R Coll Surg Engl. 2006;88(2):210–3.
10. Haylen BT, de Ridder D, Freeman RM, et al. An International Urogynecological Association (IUGA)/International Continence Society (ICS) joint report on the terminology for female pelvic floor dysfunction. Neurourol Urodyn. 2010;29(1):4–20.
11. Abrams P. Urodynamic techniques. In: Abrams P, editor. Urodynamics. 3rd ed. Bristol: Springer; 2005. p. 17–116.
12. Haylen BT, Parys BT, Anyaegbunam WI, Ashby D, West CR. Urine flow rates in male and female urodynamic patients compared with the Liverpool nomograms. Br J Urol. 1990;65(5):483–7.
13. Peterson AC, Webster GD. Urodynamic and videourodynamic evaluation of voiding dysfunction. In: Wein AJ, Novick AC, Partin AW, Peters CA, editors. Campbell-Walsh Urology, vol. 3. 9th ed. Philadelphia: Saunders-Elsevier; 2007. p. 1986–2010.

14. Kolman C, Girman CJ, Jacobsen SJ, Lieber MM. Distribution of post-void residual urine volume in randomly selected men. J Urol. 1999;161(1):122–7.
15. McGuire EJ, Woodside JR, Borden TA, Weiss RM. Prognostic value of urodynamic testing in myelodysplastic patients. J Urol. 1981;126(2):205–9.
16. Resnick NM, Yalla SV, Laurino E. The pathophysiology of urinary incontinence among institutionalized elderly persons. N Engl J Med. 1989;320(1):1–7.

Chapter 4
Medication Issues

Mary Ann Forciea

Case Presentation

Mrs. L is an 82-year-old retired university professor who presents for the evaluation of urinary incontinence of 3 years duration. She leaks urine daily, and wears "maxi pads" daily. She does experience increased leakage while playing tennis, and did note worsening during a recent upper respiratory infection. She is functionally independent, lives alone, and plays tennis weekly. Her active medical problems include hypertension, diabetes mellitus, hyperlipidemia, glaucoma, and osteoarthritis of the lumbosacral spine. Her current daily medications include: aspirin, hydrochlorthiazide, metoprolol, enalapril, metformin, simvastatin, naproxen, and pilocarpine eye drops. She asks if anything can be done to improve her continence.

General Review of Medication Issues in Older Patients

The burden of medication management is especially important in the care of older patients since they carry a disproportionate share of chronic conditions and drug therapy: while approximately 13% of the population of the US is >65 years of age, these patients purchase 33% of all prescription drugs [1]. Increasingly, conditions such as congestive heart failure and diabetes are managed with small dose of medications from a variety of classes. The potential for adverse drug events and problems with patient adherence increase as the medication burden increases. Increasingly, medication choices are included in performance management measures [2].

M.A. Forciea (✉)
Division of Geriatric Medicine, Department of Medicine, University of Pennsylvania
Health System, Philadelphia, PA 19104, USA
e-mail: forciea@mail.med.upenn.edu

T.J. Guzzo et al. (eds.), *Primer of Geriatric Urology*, DOI 10.1007/978-1-4614-4773-3_4,   33
© Springer Science+Business Media New York 2013

Optimal medication management for patients of any age follows the adage,

The correct *drug*
In the correct *dose*
For the correct *patient*
At an affordable *cost*

Treatment of older patients can require special considerations at each of these steps.

The "Correct" Drug and Dose

1. *Pharmacokinetic* considerations with age: "Start low, go slow."

The time course of action of a drug and its metabolites constitute its *pharmacokinetic* properties. These properties of drugs are usually grouped into changes in their *absorption, distribution, metabolism,* and *elimination.* Considerations in each of these four areas can be important in older patients.

a. *Absorption*

In general, few clinically significant changes in drug absorption from the GI tract are seen in older patients. More important can be drug administration factors which can influence absorption:

- Decreased gastric pH (either intrinsic or due to acid secretion blockers) may change absorption of antibiotics or vitamins
- Alterations in GI motility due to constipation, diarrhea, or medications may change absorption due to transit time alterations through various segments of bowel
- Simultaneous administration of medications can create obstacles to absorption: cations like calcium may adsorb other medication such as synthroid or fluoroquinolone antibiotics
- Parenteral tube administration of medications can be complicated by interactions with feeding solutions or by changes in motility related to osmolality changes in the feeding solutions

Cooperation among care teams especially in inpatient and nursing home settings is essential to design medication administration schedules which maximize absorption of needed medications. Consultant long-term care pharmacists can be of great assistance in this endeavor.

b *Distribution*

Drug distribution is usually expressed as a volume of distribution (V_d) with units of volume or volume per weight. Drug penetration into the body spaces and time to steady state concentration alters with aging due to age-associated body composition changes. Body fat content increases, so that lipophylic drugs have a larger volume of distribution. Drugs such as flurazepam take longer to reach steady state and require longer times for elimination.

In addition, transport factors can influence distribution. Albumin, the plasma protein most associated with drug binding, can be reduced in concentration in older patients. Reduced protein binding may result in elevated-free levels, and potentially increased toxicity. Two drugs influenced by this phenomenon are warfarin and phenytoin.

c *Metabolism*

The liver and kidneys are the two organs most associated with drug metabolism in older patients.

Liver metabolism of drugs in older patients can be reduced because of decreased hepatic blood flow and by decreased hepatic mass. In the liver, drugs are metabolized by phase I or phase II pathways. Phase I reactions include hydroxylation, oxidation, dealkylation, and reduction. Metabolites can be equipotent, less potent or more potent than the original drugs; effects can be unpredictable in older patients. Phase II reactions involve glucuronidation, conjugation, or acetylation. These metabolites are generally inactive and are less likely to contribute to toxicity.

The kidneys are actively involved in Vitamin D metabolism, converting 25-hydroxy Vitamin D to the highly active 1, 25, dihydroxy Vit D. Declines in kidney function can contribute to vit D deficiency syndromes in patients with renal failure

d *Elimination*

Terms useful in consideration of the elimination of drugs from the body are:

Clearance—the volume of plasma or serum from which a drug is removed per unit of time, L/min
Half life—time required for a drug concentration to decline by 50%
Steady state—the amount of drug entering the circulation equals the amount eliminated. Most drugs reach steady state concentration after five half lives

While liver alterations may play a role in the elimination of some drugs, most drugs and metabolites require renal involvement for elimination. While renal tubular excretion can change with aging, most attention has focused on the declines in glomerular filtration with aging. Declines in glomerular filtration can vary with individuals, and are poorly reflected in the serum creatinine. The traditional algorithm for calculating GFR (via creatinine clearance-CrCl) is the Cockcroft–Gault equation [1]:

$$\text{Creatinine Clearance} = \{(140 - \text{age}) \times \text{weight(kg)}\} / (72 \times \text{serum Cr}).$$

The value of the equation is usually reduced to 85% in women. While many electronic medical record systems report Cr Cl via the Cockcroft–Gault equation, the clinician must remember that the equation become less reliable in situations of low flow and low muscle mass which are commonly seen in older frail patients. *Whenever possible, measurement of blood levels of drugs (aminoglycosides, anticonvulsants) in older patients is the best guide to dosing levels.*

Table 4.1 Summary of pharmacokinetic changes with aging

	Age-associated change	Medication examples
Absorption	Increased possibility of drug–drug interactions in GI tract (polypharmacy)	Proton pump inhibitors and antibiotics, calcium salts and synthroid
Distribution	Increased body fat stores	Anesthetic agents-warfarin, phenytoin
	Decreased albumin concentration and drug binding	
Metabolism	Decreased liver metabolism	Benzodiazepines
Elimination	Decreased renal clearance	Aminoglycosides, anticonvulsants

Pharmacodynamics, the time course and intensity of effect can vary widely and unpredictably in older patients. Morphine can produce slightly longer pain relief in some older patients, for example. Adjustments in initial dose and dosing intervals may be required for many medications.

When initiating a new medication in an older patient, the adage "start low, go slow" remains useful: start with small initial doses, with longer dose intervals; increase dose or alter intervals as symptoms require. Table 4.1 summaries these principles.

The "Correct" Patient

Choosing the *best medication* at the right dose and dosing interval for your individual patient is the foundation of prescribing for patients of any age. In selecting a medication for an older patient, certain factors may influence the choice of an initial medication:

Effectiveness—New drugs are rarely tested in older patients due to age-based elimination from initial drug study panels. While the FDA is encouraging more inclusive criteria in patient selection for initial testing, issues of coexisting disease will likely continue to limit the inclusion of representative older patients in studies. Prescribing a newly licensed drug to older patients requires the ability of the patient and physician to identify and monitor both effectiveness and side effects in this population. Often, the choice of an established medication is safer for an older patient.

Harms:

- Adverse effects of newly licensed medications are unpredictable in older patients
- Certain classes of medications are more likely to cause an adverse effect in an older patient

   - Anticholinergic drugs may precipitate acute glaucoma, bladder outlet obstruction, bradycardias, and syncope. Donepezil prescribed for memory loss is increasingly reported as linked to bradyarrhythmias and syncope
   - Opiods will increase constipation, and may cause confusion
   - Antibiotic use may result in bacterial overgrowth colitis

Table 4.2 A sample of potentially inappropriate drugs for the elderly from the Beer's list

Medication class	Example	Rationale
Nonsteroidal anti-inflammatory agents	Naproxen	Renal failure, GI bleeding
Barbiturates	Phenobarbital	Confusion
Benzodiazepines	Chlordiazepoxide, diazepam	Prolonged sedation
Hypnotics	Diphenhydramine, flurazepam	Confusion, prolonged sedation
Muscle relaxants	Cyclobenzaprine, methocarbamol	Anticholinergic effects
Pain relievers	Meperidine, propoxyphene	Confusion, minimal benefit
Antihypertensives	Clonidine	Bradycardia, orthostatic hypotension

A commonly used source of medications to be potentially avoided in older adults is the "Beers list" [3, 4]. A sample of drugs appearing on the list with rationale appears in Table 4.2. If an individual patient has a strong preference for a medication on the Beer's list, chart documentation of the rational should be provided.

- Drug–drug interactions are more likely due to the increased average number of medications taken by older patients.

Cost—Many older patients are on limited income, and take multiple medications. Most seniors are now using insurance plans with established formularies to help pay for medications; either Medicare "Part D" plans or state Medicaid formularies. Established medications are more likely to be included in these formularies and require less staff time with preauthorization for use.

Adherence: "Affordable Cost" and Other Factors

Older patients may experience special barriers to filling prescriptions and continuing medications as prescribed. Studies have shown that approximately 50% of older patients have adherence issues with at least one medication. Complicating things further, patients may be non-adherent with one medication and adherent with others [5]!

Cost—Pharmacy data suggests that as many as 40% of prescriptions are never "picked-up" by patients. Cost is a major factor in this initial loss of adherence, as well as with ongoing care. As mentioned above, older patients are on a fixed income, and use insurance-based formularies for medications payment. Many of these insurance plans require co-payments for medications. With increasing numbers of prescribed medications, the co-payment amounts may become limiting. Prescribing generic forms of medications whenever possible will aid in this aspect of care.

Literacy—Standard prescription labels are too small for many older patients to read, and use medical words which are poorly understood. Some of the larger chain store pharmacies have instituted larger print, more legible labeling practices. Physician offices can assist by providing large print medication lists with instructions for patients at the time of visits.

Manual dexterity—"Child proof" bottles can be extremely difficult for older patients to open. This can result in patients removing pills from their original bottles, which can increase medication confusion. Non-childproof bottles can be ordered for older patients, with cautions if young children are in the home. A wide variety of "pill boxes" which are preloaded by family members or nursing personnel are available. Some of these dispensers are automated, and dispense at a fixed time of day with an alert signal for the patient. Inhaled medications should be ordered with a spacer or nebulizer if the patient cannot demonstrate good multi-dose inhaler technique in the office. Some pharmacies will dispense pills in "blister packs" with all the pills for a given time of day grouped together in a plastic blister. The patient or caregiver opens the blister rather than opening several bottles.

Adverse Events of Medications in Older Patients

It has been estimated that 20% of all Emergency Department visits by older patients are related to adverse effects of medications. In addition to the risks of individual medications mentioned above, and to drug–drug interactions in patients on multiple medications, older patients have additional risks of adverse effects:

- Vision limitations interfere with prescription label reading and pill identification
- Complex medication administration regimen can be difficult to understand or implement
- Lack of understanding about indication for individual medications can lead to errors
- Cognitive impairment which impacts all of the above. Many of these cognitive impairments are mild enough to escape identification on brief medical encounters, but substantial enough to interfere with medication adherence
- In Nursing Home settings, multiple dosing interval schedules ("TID" is not the same as "every 8 h" for instance), may result in multiple medication nursing passes, and increased opportunities for errors

Clearly written prescriptions which include indication for use and the simplest dosing regimen possible will aid with adherence in any setting. Nursing home physicians should work with pharmacy and nursing staff to streamline medication administration wherever possible.

On occasion, patients admitted to a hospital or nursing home with hypertension or diabetes develop complications such as hypotension or hypoglycemia within the first 48 h of admission. Consideration of prior adherence issues at home with medications may be in order before new diagnostic work-ups are initiated. Patients may NOT, in fact, have been taking their medications as ordered. When medications are ordered from record-based lists and administered by nursing staff, overmedication may result. *Patients or caregivers should be politely but firmly questioned about ACTUAL medications and dosing regimen in use at home.*

Transitions of Care Medication Issues

At discharge from the acute care hospital or nursing home, special care should be taken in the ordering and review of discharge medications [2, 6]. Any deviation from admission medications should be carefully explained. In many instances, hospital formulary composition necessitates changes in medication within a class during the admission. Whenever possible, patients should be returned to their original medication (with which they are familiar and likely have a supply at home), or have careful instructions about in-class medication changes. The risk of duplicate medication without these precautions is high. Returning the patient to a preexisting medication list also alleviates the need to check with the patient's drug plan formulary for availability since the patient had been receiving supplies of baseline medications.

For patients experiencing a major change in function, transfer or admission to a long-term care facility may offer a chance for reconsideration of need for medication [4]. Does the patient's current life expectancy justify ongoing medication? Does the medication fit with the patient's current goals of care?

Urinary Incontinence (UI): Medical Management Options

Medications for Urinary Incontinence

Most of the medications available for UI address urge incontinence, and have been shown to be effective in older patients. The antimuscarinic agents differ in anticholinergic potency and metabolism. Table 4.3 lists the commonly available choices. Contraindications to the use of antimuscarinic agents in older patients are:

- A history of urinary retention
- Impaired gastric emptying
- Narrow angle glaucoma

Antimuscarinic agents can be safe in older patients if started at the lowest doses and titrated up as needed and with monitoring. Evaluation of post-void residual urine volume should be considered in those patients who develop increased incontinence on this class of medication, reflecting possible overflow incontinence. Long-term use of this class of medication can be associated with xerostomia, leading to increased dental caries and tooth loss. An increase in confusion may also be seen after initiation of antimuscarinic agents. This risk of confusion is especially strong in patients who are receiving anticholinergic medications such as donepezil for dementia. Little evidence suggests that one member of the class is superior to another in an individual patient. Choice of agent should depend on adverse event profile, drug interactions, dosing regimen, and cost. Failure of one agent should not preclude a trial of another member of the class.

Table 4.3 Medications available for UI in older patients

Antimuscarinic agents
Oxybutinin (as immediate release, extended release, or patch) 2.5 mg twice daily, max 5 mg twice daily
Tolteridine (immediate or extended release) 1 mg twice daily, max 2 mg twice daily, metabolism CYP 3A4
Trospium 20 mg/day
Darifenacin 7.5 mg/day, max 15 mg/day; liver metabolism, CYP3A4
Solifenacin 5 mg/day, max 10 mg/day metabolized in liver, CYP 450:3A4 substrate
Topical estrogen

Topical estrogen may be useful in stress incontinence in postmenopausal women due to improvements in vaginal mucous production.

Behavioral Therapy for Urinary Incontinence

Non-pharmacologic alternatives to the treatment of some urologic problems are available and useful for older patients [7].

Urinary Incontinence treatments offer the widest array of behavioral approaches (see also Chap. 7).

Lifestyle modifications-Alterations in daily practices may alleviate the symptoms of urinary incontinence in many patients. Simple adjustments, such as the timing of diuretic administration (moving a second dose from 8 PM to 4 PM) may alleviate nocturia with leaking. Certain foods can be bladder irritants: spicy foods, citrus fruits, and artificial sweeteners. Caffeine is both a diuretic and a smooth muscle irritant. Food diaries can allow individual patients to track dietary exposures and bladder contraction related urinary leakage. Chronic constipation may contribute to urinary incontinence. Smoking can lead to incontinence due to both increased coughing, and to the bladder contractions associated with nicotine exposure. Weight reduction in morbidly obese women has been shown to result in decreased symptoms of urinary incontinence.

Kegel exercises—Patients with stress urinary incontinence related to pelvic muscle relaxation can benefit from a program of pelvic muscle exercise. These exercises were first described by Dr Arnold Kegel in 1948 [8]. Patients (women and post-prostatectomy men) are taught to:

- Identify pelvic floor muscles—usually taught by asking the patient to contract the rectal muscles used to prevent expelling flatus
- Intentionally contract these pelvic floor muscles, and sustain the contraction for from 2 to 5 s. Patients gradually increase the time of the longer contractions to 10 s
- Repeat these brief and more sustained contractions in sets of 10–30 repetitions three times daily. Patients should rotate positions to include lying, seated, and standing postures

Successful Kegel exercise muscle strengthening has been demonstrated to improve urinary incontinence in women and men, is free (after the original instruction), has no drug interactions, and can improve the older patient's sense of empowerment. Strong evidence supports the efficacy of pelvic floor muscle exercise programs for the prevention and treatment of incontinence. Preoperative training in Kegel exercises can reduce post-prostatectomy incontinence.

Bladder training programs—A variety of techniques are available which involve voiding at intervals. Presumably, intentional emptying of the bladder before volume-related continence loss will reduce incontinence. Most of these scheduling programs are followed during waking hours only. These techniques include:

- *Scheduled voiding*—Patients are taught (or reminded) to toilet on a fixed schedule (often every 3 h). While convenient for nursing staff in facilities or for caregivers, the fixed intervals may not match individual patient needs
- *Habit training*—After completion of a voiding diary, a schedule of toileting is developed for an individual patient (perhaps 30 min after breakfast, 2 h later, and then 3 h intervals)
- *Prompted voiding*—This technique can be used by caregivers of patients with dementia. After completion of a voiding diary, patients are asked about wetness or dryness at determined intervals. If dry, they are offered toilet opportunities and/or assistance. Positive feedback for dryness is provided
- *Bladder retraining*—For cognitively intact patients who are motivated to decrease incontinence episodes, an adjustable voiding regimen can be developed. Patients are educated about techniques to reduce urge-associated voiding to prolong intervals between voids. These techniques can include distraction and relaxation strategies. As control increases, intervals between voids are increased

Physical Rehabilitation Techniques—Electrical or magnetic stimulation of the bladder has been proposed in the treatment of urinary incontinence. A review of randomized controlled trials of both techniques has showed limited evidence that these techniques improved continence more than sham controls or pelvic floor muscle training. Biofeedback techniques can improve awareness of pelvic floor muscle contractions, and serve as an adjunct to pelvic floor muscle (Kegel) training. In biofeedback, electrodes are placed on the skin or inside the vagina and rectum. Indices of muscle contraction strength and endurance can be used to help design individualized programs of exercise. The use of weighted vaginal cones can also improve pelvic floor muscle strength. Women are taught the routines of insertion/removal and cleaning between uses. Women insert the lighted cone and retain it for up to 15 min twice daily. As pelvic muscle strength improves, heavier cones are inserted. The cones are highly acceptable to some patients, but not all. While some evidence exists as to the efficacy of cones, little evidence shows them to be superior to Kegel exercises alone.

Case Presentation Return

After checking for a urinary tract infection and counseling about avoidance of caffeine, Mrs. L should be instructed in pelvic floor muscle (Kegel) exercises. If she has difficulty identifying the appropriate muscles, biofeedback could be included in her treatment plan. She might also benefit from bladder retraining to increase the time between voluntary voids. If her symptoms of urinary incontinence persist, she could begin a trial of oxybutinin.

References

1. Semla TP. Pharmacotherapy. In: Pacala JT, Sullivan GM, editors. Geriatric review syllabus: a core curriculum in geriatric medicine. 7th ed. New York: American Geriatrics Society; 2010. p. 82–91.
2. Shrank WH, Polinski JM, Avorn J. Quality indicators for medication use in vulnerable elders. J Am Geriatr Soc. 2007;55:S373–82.
3. Fick DM, Cooper JW, Wade WE, Waller JL, Maclean JR, Beers MH. Updating the Beers criteria for potentially inappropriate medication use in older adults: results of a US consensus panel of experts. Arch Intern Med. 2003;163:2716–24.
4. Holmes HM, Hayley DC, Alexander GC, Sachs GA. Reconsidering medication appropriateness for patients late in life. Arch Intern Med. 2006;166:605–9.
5. Steinman MA, Hanlon JT. Managing medication in clinically complex elders. JAMA. 2010;304:1592–601.
6. Meeks TW, Culberson JW, Horton MS. Medications in long-term care: when less is more. Clin Geriatr Med. 2011;27:1717–9.
7. Newman DK, Wein AJ. Managing and treating urinary incontinence. 2nd ed. Baltimore: Health Professions Press; 2009.
8. Kegel AH. Progressive resistance exercise in the functional restoration of the perineal muscles. Am J Obst Gynec. 1948;56(2):238–48.

Chapter 5
Perioperative Care of the Geriatric Urology Patient

Eugene J. Pietzak and Thomas J. Guzzo

Introduction

Approximately half of all urologic surgeries in the United States are performed in patients 65 years of age or older [1].It is also estimated that by the year 2030, 20% of the United States population with be greater than 75 years old [2]. With the increasing elderly population worldwide, the proportion of patients in this age group presenting for surgery on an annual basis will certainly increase. With proper patient selection, careful planning, and optimal perioperative management, surgery can be safely performed in elderly patients with comparable risk to younger individuals [3]. Although there has been significant improvement over the last few decades in surgical technology and anesthesia delivery, the elderly continue to represent a unique and challenging population of surgical patients.

Preoperative Assessment

While chronologic age should never be considered a contraindication to even elective surgery, it is important to recognize that elderly patients are at increased risk for a number of perioperative complications compared to younger patients who undergo similar surgical procedures [4]. The increased risk of complications for the geriatric

E.J. Pietzak · T.J. Guzzo (✉)
Department of Surgery, Division of Urology, Perelman Center for Advanced Medicine,
Hospital of the University of Pennsylvania, Philadelphia, PA 19104, USA
e-mail: Eugene.pietzak@uphs.upenn.edu; thomas.guzzo@uphs.upenn.edu

T.J. Guzzo et al. (eds.), *Primer of Geriatric Urology*, DOI 10.1007/978-1-4614-4773-3_5,   43
© Springer Science+Business Media New York 2013

surgical patient is multi-factorial [5]. Elderly patients are more likely than younger patients to have more co-morbidities, more medications, and an impaired functional status [5, 6]. Geriatric patients are often able to handle the initial stress of surgery but some may lack the reserve to handle a complication [7], thus leading to worse outcomes [8]. An estimated 20% of patients older than 80 years of age who undergo noncardiac surgery will experience a postoperative complication, placing them at greater risk of death [9]. Similarly, a retrospective review of the American College of Surgeons National Surgical Quality Improvement Program database revealed that elderly patients undergoing gastrointestinal surgery have significantly higher rates of morbidity and mortality, even when adjusted for preoperative co-morbidities [10].

While a routine history and physical is standard for any patient prior to a surgical procedure, a detailed assessment of co-morbid conditions, medication history, nutritional status, and functional status is essential to minimize the risk of complications for elderly patients.

While taking a history, it is important to recognize that elderly patients may be hard of hearing, have poor memory, and may minimize symptoms out of fear of loss of independence [11]. Up to 40% of outpatients with cognitive impairment seen may not have the diagnosis of dementia documented in their chart [12]. Geriatric patients may also have a delay in presentation and present with more severe conditions [11].

The goal of the preoperative assessment is to evaluate for perioperative risk and to identify problems that can be optimized before surgery. It is during the preoperative assessment that discussion over postoperative care should begin to ensure an appropriate postoperative discharge plan is in place.

Medical Co-morbidities

Elderly patients typically have more medical conditions than that of younger surgical patients. Common medical problems seen in the elderly include dementia, Chronic Obstructive Pulmonary Disease (COPD), diabetes, coronary artery disease (CAD), congestive heart failure, and hypertension. The presence, as well as severity, of co-morbidity can be a valuable predictor of postoperative outcome for many urological procedures [13–15]. As one might expect, the presence of co-morbid conditions has been shown to be a more useful predictor of perioperative outcomes than chronologic age alone [16].

Medications

A thorough review of current medications is important as 40% of individuals 65 years or older are on five or more medications [17]. It is not uncommon for elderly patients to have more than one doctor prescribing them medications.

Additionally, medications targeting the cardiovascular system and central nervous system are common prescriptions in this age group. Polypharmacy obviously complicates perioperative management and often requires consultation and coordination with other specialists.

Knowledge of an elderly patient's medication history can reduce the potential for drug interactions. Known allergies and any previous adverse reactions should be sought. Any over-the-counter drugs, herbal, or dietary supplements should also be obtained. Older patients are more likely to be taking anti-coagulants, aspirin, and nonsteriodal anti-inflammatory drugs which need to be stopped for many procedures. Although there is no consensus on optimal perioperative management for these medications, the goal is to minimize the window of time which the patient is at increased risk for thrombosis while balancing the increased risk of perioperative bleeding.

Nutritional Status

The detrimental impact of malnourishment is easily underappreciated by surgeons. Although definitions of malnourishment vary between studies, the rate of malnourishment in urology patients is estimated at around 16–21% [18, 19]. Malnourishment increases with age and can result from multiple factors, including underlying co-morbidities, poor dentition, poor functional status, and medications that alter digestion, absorption, appetite, taste, and smell [20, 21].

Malnourishment is a significant risk factor for postoperative complications following urologic surgery [22]. This is especially true for patients undergoing radical urologic surgeries, where malnourishment may be the strongest risk factor for morbidity and mortality [19, 23]. These findings are consistent with previous literature from Gibbs et al. which showed that low preoperative albumin is the strongest predictor of morbidity and mortality in major noncardiac surgery [24]. However, serum albumin levels do not just reflect an inadequate dietary intake, but may be affected by co-morbidities, inflammatory cytokines, and medications [18, 25, 26].

Regardless, it is clear that adequate nutrients are required for proper surgical wound healing and recovery from the catabolic stress of surgery [27–30]. Total Parental Nutrition (TPN) has been used, but, offers minimal benefit to surgical patients and increases infectious risk [31, 32]. Interventions such as jejunostomy and gastrostomy feedings have been tried but are highly invasive and not without complications [33]. Early postoperative oral feedings have been shown to shorten length of hospital stay [34], however, it offers little benefit to patients who are malnourished prior to surgery. Preoperative oral nutritional supplementation has been shown to decrease complications in several surgical fields, offering promise for improving outcomes in undernourished surgical patients [35, 36]. The role for preoperative oral supplementation is still under investigation for urologic surgery.

Related to malnourishment is the clinical entity of sarcopenia. The criteria of sarcopenia is analogous to that of osteoporosis; muscle mass that is two standard deviations below the mean for healthy young reference populations [37]. It is estimated that approximately 20–30% of the population between 70 and 80 years old have sarcopenia [38]. From the second to eighth decade of life, almost half of all muscle mass is lost [39]. Muscle loss results from physical inactivity that frequently occurs with aging, as well as, inflammatory-induced atrophy from increasing co-morbidities [37]. The presence of sarcopenia portends a poor prognosis overall and is associated with significant postoperative morbidity and mortality [40, 41].

Although not a linear relationship between muscle mass and function, they are closely associated. Indices of muscular function, such as gait speed and grip strength, are better at predicting survival and adverse outcomes [42–44]. Loss of muscle mass in the elderly not only negatively impacts functional levels but also cardiopulmonary function, glucose management, and levels of amino acids needed for recovery from surgery [37].

The ratio of muscle to fat is roughly 2:1 for healthy young men, but, this ratio is reversed in the elderly [37]. So, as muscle mass decreases with age, fat mass increases. This can result in a similar BMI despite vastly different body compositions as one ages. If extreme, sarcopenic obesity can occur [45]. The coexistence of sacropenia and obesity in the same individual may result in worse morbidity and mortality than if either condition was present alone [46].

Obesity in elderly patients, even in the absence of sarcopenia, is associated with significant disability and negatively impacts quality of life [47]. Obesity places all surgical patients, regardless of age, at risk for complications [48]. Although weight loss prior to planned surgery may benefit these patients, careful attention is needed for calorie restriction in the elderly to avoid inadequate intake of essential nutrients resulting in malnourishment.

Functional Status

An overall assessment of the geriatric patient's functional status is paramount. Functional state tends to decrease with age, leaving elderly patients with less physiologic reserve to recover from the stress of surgery and to compensate for complications [5, 7]. Functional status includes all physical and cognitive behaviors, which are necessary to maintain independent activities of daily living (ADL) [5]. A patient's overall functional status is often determined by assessing their ability to perform both ADL and instrumental ADL [5]. Inability to complete ADLs is associated with an increased risk of postoperative morbidity and mortality [5, 49]. Seymour and Pringle demonstrated that the inability to leave home by one's own efforts at least twice a week was independently associated with a higher risk of major postoperative surgical complications [50]. Functional status is also associated with an increased need for intensive rehabilitation services following surgery [51], including need for nursing facilities upon discharge. Lack of independence on ADLs is also a significant risk factor for readmissions following surgery [49]. Objective measures of functional status, such as gait speed, have also been shown to predict length of hospital stay and discharge status for elderly patients admitted to a geriatric hospital unit [52].

Global Assessment

Recently, the comprehensive geriatric assessment (CGA) has been shown to be a useful predictor of perioperative complications in elderly patients [53]. The CGA allows for a more global gauge of physiologic health as opposed to relying on the chronologic age of a patient. The CGA considers functional status, co-morbid conditions, cognitive functions, psychological state, social support, nutritional status, and geriatric syndromes in the overall assessment of an elderly patient's status [54]. It can therefore act as a robust indicator of the overall ability of an elderly individual to tolerate a major operative procedure. The CGA prior to surgical intervention may improve functional status postoperatively as well as reduce hospital and nursing home stays, potentially decreasing overall costs [55].

Preoperative Risk Assessment

Studies in both the oncologic and non-oncologic setting have demonstrated the CGA to be a valuable preoperative risk assessment tool for elderly patients [5, 55]. However, the American Society of Anesthesiologists Classification (ASA) is the most common system used for stratification of surgical risk and nearly every patient taken to the operating room is assigned an ASA score [56]. ASA physical status score is an excellent predictor of mortality for elderly patients undergoing prostatectomy [56]. Although, ASA is the most widely used preoperative risk assessment, it does not have perfect predictive ability. ASA has been combined with emergency status and procedural risk to develop a Surgical Mortality Probability Model to estimate the 30 day all-cause mortality after surgery [57]. Other co-morbidity scores exist when contemplating surgical risk, including the Charlson Comorbidity Index (CCI) and the Cumulative Illness Rating Scale for Geriatrics (CIRS-G) [55]. CCI has been widely used in urologic literature for both oncologic and non-oncologic surgery [14, 58, 59]. However CCI is limited because it does not factor in the severity of a given co-morbidity. CIRS-G rates the burden of physical illness and should take less than 10 min to complete [60, 61]. Preoperative assessment in elderly cancer patients (PACE) is a comprehensive surgical assessment tool that combines CGA, fatigue level, performance status, and the anesthesiologist's evaluation of operative risk [62]. The team that developed PACE believes it should be used routinely in assessing elderly cancer patients for surgery [62]. Also, whenever assessing geriatric patients for surgery it is important to evaluate for frailty [63, 64]. If frailty is identified it may be an indication that medical optimization may be needed prior to surgery [65].

Preoperative Testing

The purpose of preoperative testing is to assess the severity of a known medical condition and to detect unsuspected abnormalities [66]. While routine labs are commonly performed, there is little evidence to support this practice [66]. Most abnormalities would be predicted by history and physical exam and it is rare for abnormal findings to change perioperative care [67, 68]. Considering preoperative testing accounts for an estimated 3–30 billion dollars in annual healthcare costs for the United States [69, 70], some advocate not ordering tests based on age alone, but based on the individual patient and the planned surgery [71].

For cardiac risk stratification, exercise tolerance is a strong independent predictor for postoperative cardiovascular complications [72]. The inability to elevate heart rate above 99 beats per minute during 2 min of exercise, while on a supine bike is predictive of both cardiac and pulmonary complications [73, 74]. Most patients who can exercise greater than four metabolic equivalent of task (e.g., walking at a very brisk pace or carrying clubs while golfing) are at very low risk for cardiopulmonary complications and may not need preoperative cardiac clearance [75]. Several cardiac risk indices exist for stratification of noncardiac surgery, the most widely used is the Revised Cardiac Risk Index [76–79]. Routine electrocardiogram (ECG) is often obtain for all elderly patients, however ECG is poor at detecting existing CAD and predicting postoperative cardiac complications [80, 81]. Regardless, a preoperative ECG can be obtained to provide a baseline for comparison in case of any postoperative event.

Patients with poor overall health status, extensive smoking history, COPD, asthma, and obstructive sleep apnea are at greatest risk for pulmonary complications [75, 82]. A baseline arterial blood gas may be helpful for managing these patients. Smoking is a strong risk factor that is modifiable. Smoking cessation has a physiologic benefit after only 48 h, however, it may take at least 6–8 weeks for a decrease in pulmonary complications to occur [83]. Although all patients should be counseled by their physicians to quit smoking, this is especially true for patients with a history of bladder cancer. Along with all the known health benefits of smoking cessation, continued smoking is associated with an increased risk of recurrence and disease progression in bladder cancer [84–86]. Patients are often unaware of the association between smoking and bladder cancer [87]. Unfortunately, urologists have done a poor job at appropriately counseling these patients on smoking cessation [88].

Anesthetic Considerations in the Elderly

As with surgical planning, the anesthetic plan for geriatric patients is often more complicated than for younger patients. This complexity results from the increased number of co-morbidities, various medications, poor nutrition, worse functional status, and also from the detrimental impact aging has on physiologic function. The cardiac, pulmonary, and renal systems all undergo changes with aging that needs to be taken into account when considering a particular anesthetic approach in the elderly.

Cardiac changes frequently found in the elderly patient include a lower sensitivity to beta-adrenergic modulation, altered calcium regulation, and an overall reduction in ejection fraction [89, 90]. Limited cardiac reserve results in a higher risk of hypotension at the time of general anesthetic induction [91]. Maximal heart rate also declines with age resulting in a diminished ability to increase heart rate in response to hypovolemia, hypotension, or hypoxia [4, 91, 92]. Additionally, many elderly surgical patients will have occult CAD, prompting a low threshold for preoperative cardiac evaluation for elective procedures [4]. Diastolic dysfunction is also common in the elderly, and if severe may require arterial pressure monitoring or intra-operative transesophageal echocardiogram monitoring [93].

Pulmonary changes that accompany aging include decreased elasticity of lung tissue and weakened respiratory musculature [91]. Decreased pulmonary elasticity places patients at higher risk of small airway collapse with anesthesia which ultimately results in less efficient gas exchange from decreased alveolar surface area [91].

Renal function and glomerular filtration rate (GFR) also decline with age [94]. Serum creatinine is not a good surrogate for GFR as it often overestimates renal function in this patient population since elderly patients have less muscle mass to produce creatinine. When dosing medications, the overestimations of GFR must take into account. Many renally excreted medications, such as pancurium, may need to be avoided in elderly patients. Very careful attention must be given to fluid balance to minimize complications. Excessive intravenous fluids can easily result in prolonged mechanical ventilation in the geriatric population [95]. Further complicating fluid balance management is the decreased renal concentrating ability and thirst perception that often occurs with aging. This can result in dehydration and electrolyte abnormalities [11].

Changes in body composition also alter the distribution, metabolism, and elimination of drugs [4]. With aging, lean body mass, and total body water decreases while body fat increases [96]. As a consequence, volume of distribution from water-soluble drugs decreases leading to increased concentrations of these drugs. Fat soluble drugs will have a prolonged action. Hepatic metabolism of drugs also decreases with age, which can contribute to prolonged drug effects [97]. Appropriate adjustments in anesthetic medications must be done to account for the changes in pharmacokinetics and pharmacodynamics with aging.

The choice of anesthetic modality (general or regional) should be selected on a case by case basis taking into account both the operative approach and the patient's ability to tolerate various forms of anesthesia. Regional anesthesia is thought to have a lower incidence of pulmonary complication [4]. Decreased airway reflexes that occur with aging may partially explain this from general anesthesia leaving the patient more prone to aspiration [98]. However, there is no difference in mortality between general and regional [4]. Also, the initial concerns of an association between postoperative cognitive dysfunction and general anesthesia have been proven to be unfounded [4].

Intra-Operative Considerations

Appropriate positioning and padding is important for the safety of all patients, but especially for the elderly [99]. With aging there is often a reduction in the thickness of the epidermis and subcutaneous tissues, which increases the risk of pressure ulcers and the likelihood of nerve compression [100, 101]. Contributing to this is reduced skin elasticity, which increases the likelihood of damage. It is essential that all pressure points are placed on soft padding [100]. This is especially true if any artificial joints are present as there can be altered sensation and circulation in those area.

Elderly patients are also less mobile and relatively inflexible compared to younger patients. The prevalence of osteoarthritis is almost 50% in people 80 years or older [102]. Special care must be taken with positioning and transferring patients with osteoporosis to reduce the risk of iatrogenic fractures. Modifications in the usual procedure position may need to be made for elderly patients. Agreement over the best position and padding should be reached between the surgical team, anesthesiologists, and nursing staff prior to beginning the surgery. For medico-legal purposes, documentation of protective measures should be done.

Caution should be used when putting elderly patients in trendelenburg, especially at steep angles. There is evidence that steep trendenlenburg may increase intraocular pressure which places patients with glaucoma at risk for vision loss [103]. Also trendelenburg position decreases ventilation and ventricular filling, which may increase the risk of cardiopulmonary complications [104].

Surgical Approach

Laparoscopic surgery may have some advantages over an open approach for elderly patients [3]. The typical quicker overall convalescence, lower narcotic requirements, shorter length of hospital stay, and earlier resumption of diet associated with laparoscopy can greatly benefit the geriatric patient [105, 106]. This must be balanced with the potential for longer surgical time with certain laparoscopic procedures [107]. Increased surgical time is associated with cognitive dysfunction in the elderly [108], and is associated with higher rate of pulmonary complications [109]. Also, some laparoscopic procedures have a higher rate of intra-operative complications compared to an open approach [106, 109]. Although, age alone does not put a patient at a higher risk for a laparoscopic complication, elderly patients are less equipped to handle a complication when they do occur [15]. However, the use of robotic assistance may lead to a decrease in the rate of complications [110]. Ultimately, selection of the surgical approach should be based on the individual patient and the comfort of the surgeon.

Reducing Risk of Intra-Operative Complications

The rate of cardiovascular complication for urologic surgery is at least 2% [111]. Between 10 and 40% of all perioperative deaths are secondary to myocardial infarction [112]. Several perioperative pharmacologic interventions have been used to reduce the risk of cardiac complications. Prophaylatic beta-blockade reduces myocardial demand and prevents an exaggerated postoperative sympathetic response [113, 114]. To avoid the risk of hypotension, stroke, and mortality, lower doses of beta-blockers should be used and then titrated over time [115, 116]. Perioperative statins have also been used given their ability to stabilize coronary plaque and decrease inflammation [117]. Retrospective studies have shown a 38–59% reduction in morality with statins [118], but no statistical significant difference was seen in a recent randomized control study comparing fluvastatin to placebo [112]. Clinicians must also be aware that abrupt discontinuation of statins, such as being NPO after surgery, can result in a paradoxical withdrawal state that leads to worse cardiovascular outcomes [119]. Interestingly, a recent systemic review has suggested that statins may also reduce the rate of gastrointestinal and infectious complications after abdominal surgery [120]. However, prospective trials are needed before any conclusions can be reached.

Continuation of aspirin and other anti-platelet medications in the perioperative period can significantly reduce the risk of cardiovascular complications [121], but this needs to be balanced against the increased risk of bleeding. In general, patients with cardiac stents should be continued on aspirin unless bleeding risk is too great [122]. Patients on aspirin for primary prevention of acute coronary syndrome, who are at a low risk of perioperative cardiac complications, can usually have their aspirin held a week prior to the surgery [122].

It is generally recommended that perioperative glucose levels be maintained at around 110 mg/dl to avoid perioperative complications [123]. Although this glucose target may need to be shifted upwards for certain individuals at greater risk of hypoglycemia from treatment with insulin [124]. Reducing preoperative fasting time can also reduce the risk of hypoglycemia [125]. Preoperative carbohydrate-based drinks that are taken up to 2 h before surgery improves insulin sensitivity, preserves structural proteins, and improves patient comfort [126].

Perioperative hypothermia is a common occurrence in the operating room that must be avoided in geriatric patients [127]. Hypothermia depresses heart function and prolongs recovery from anesthesia [128]. Perioperative hypothermia is also associated with poor wound healing, increased infections, and discomfort [129]. Elderly patients also have more difficulty regulating their body temperature [129]. Hypothermia often results from a cool ambient temperature and use of cold intravenous fluids, especially blood product transfusions [128]. These effects can be minimized by forced-air warming [127].

Postoperative Management

There has been recent interest in the development of objective measures to assist surgeons in postoperative decision-making [130]. Since the elderly handle anesthetics differently than younger patients, the surgeon should discuss with the anesthesia team the plans for discharging or admitting an elderly patient from the post-anesthesia care unit, even if it was a short uneventful procedure [131, 132]. While discharge criteria following ambulatory surgery has existed for several decades [133], only recently has attention been given to finding an accurate objective postoperative assessment tool for major surgeries [130]. Determining risk for postoperative complications is useful for deciding on level of care needs [134]. Similar to the selection of surgical candidates, age alone should not be the sole determinant for admission to the intensive care unit [135, 136]. The Physiological and Operative Severity Score for the enUmeration of Mortality and morbidity (POSSUM) and the Acute Physiology and Chronic Health Evaluation (APACHE II) scores are commonly used predictors of postoperative risk based on their physiology. However both the POSSUM and APACHE II scores are complicated calculations that are not always practical. The Surgical APGAR score is a simpler predictor of complication, using three intra-operative measures; maximal heart rate, lowest mean arterial pressure, and estimated blood loss [134]. A modified version of the Surgical APGAR has been described for radical cystectomy patients [137]. Efforts to improve the predictive ability of these risk scores will likely focus on customizing them to specific procedures and patient populations [138]. These objective measures will likely become of increasing importance in high risk patients, such as the elderly.

Interest in postoperative clinical care pathways for many major urologic procedures has also increased recently [139, 140]. Clinical pathways provide a framework to optimize care to improve outcomes while being more cost-effective. While these clinical pathways can be applied to the geriatric population, some modifications may be needed [141].

Patients should be restarted on their home medications as soon as it is safe from a surgical standpoint. Particularly those patients on neurologic or cardiac medications. For example, even a few hours without levodopa can cause a return of Parkinson's Disease symptoms [142].

Pulmonary complications are common cause of morbidity for the elderly. Postoperative functional residual capacity can decrease by up to 70% and remain depressed for 1 week after surgery [4]. This could be improved with lung expansion by encouraging incentive spirometry, coughing, and deep breathing exercises. Preoperative education on spirometry and coughing may improve the effectiveness of these interventions [143].

Another strategy to decrease the risk of pulmonary complication is early ambulation, which improves ventilation and secretion clearance [144]. Early ambulation may also hasten return of bowel function and prevent postoperative ileus [145]. It is critical to limit bed rest for elderly patients to avoid de-conditioning of muscles, which could result in a loss of independence and need for discharge services [146].

Early ambulation also decreases the risk of Deep Venous Thrombosis (DVT) and Pulmonary Embolism (PE) from developing [147]. Along with sequential compression devices, another cornerstone of DVT/PE prevention is pharmacologic prophylaxis with heparin or low molecular weight heparin for select patients [147]. Unfortunately, adherence rates with pharmacologic prophylaxis in perioperative patients are suboptimal [148]. Urologists should be aware of the American Urologic Association's best practice statement for venous thromboembolism prevention, and follow accordingly [149].

Traditionally, postoperative oral feedings were not begun until the subjective return of bowel function due to surgeon's fear of postoperative ileus or anastomatic disruption [150]. This dogma has been challenged, and numerous studies have shown a benefit to early oral feedings, even in the setting of recent intestinal anastomosis [34, 150]. Geriatric patients would particularly benefit from early intake of nutrients to assist in postsurgical recovery.

Early resumption of oral intake also reduces the risk of electrolyte and fluid imbalances that elderly patients are more prone to [151]. Maintenance of homeostasis is complicated by the physiologic changes of aging such as GFR reduction and changes in neurohormonal regulation of electrolytes and water, which can be stressed during the perioperative period [151]. Fluid management for the elderly should begin before surgery with consideration of a shortened preoperative fast. Evidence supports a reduction of fasting time improves outcomes without increasing anesthesia risk [33, 152]. However this should be discussed with the anesthesia team before hand.

Postoperative pain is an important issue for elderly patients. With aging there is a reduction in the efficacy of endogenous analgesic systems [153]. However pain is often undertreated in the elderly, likely from the clinician's underestimation of pain and their fear of adverse events. Given the decreased drug metabolism and clearance in the elderly, narcotics and sedatives should be given with caution. However undertreatment of pain not only leads to unnecessary patient suffering, but also increases the risk of postoperative delirium [154]. The use of patient-controlled analgesia has been used successfully in the postsurgical geriatric population to provide adequate pain control that is titrated to a safe level [155, 156]. To further reduce the need for opioids, a multimodal analgesia approach with epidurals, acetaminophen, and NSAIDs should be used [157]. A patient-controlled analgesia epidural with local anesthesia not only achieves effective pain control, but reduces systemic opioid consumption, improves mental status, and bowel activity [156].

Special Considerations for the Elderly After Surgery

Delirium is a common underappreciated complication in the postoperative geriatric population. Delirium is associated with increased morbidity, functional decline, and greater length of hospital stay [158]. It increases the overall cost of hospitalization, and increases resource utilization by increasing need for inpatient nursing care and nursing home placement at time of discharge. Most importantly delirium is associated with high rates of mortality [158, 159]. The rate of delirium after major urologic abdominal surgery is estimated to be between 11 and 21% [3], however delirium is often under-recognized by nurses and physicians [160, 161].

Prevention of delirium begins with the elimination of unnecessary drugs, since they are the most common iatrogenic cause of delirium. Sedatives, narcotics, and anti-cholinergic medications are common offenders [158]. Pain control, oxygen levels, electrolytes, and fluid balance should be optimized [75]. Patients should be provided their glasses and hearing aids if needed. The patient's room should be well lit with an appropriate level of sensory stimulation.

Risk factors for postoperative delirium include age, dehydration, electrolytes abnormalities, immobilization, and preoperative dementia [75]. For a patient at high risk, a consultation with a geriatrician should be considered. A randomized control study on elderly patients with hip fractures showed that a proactive geriatrics consultation reduced the rate of delirium from 50 to 32% [162]. The severity of these episodes was also decreased. If delirium does develop the use of restraints should be avoided. Also, delirium may be a symptom of another cause, such as an infection or myocardial infarction, which should be ruled out [75].

Geriatric patients are at greater risk for aspiration due to decreased oropharynx protective reflexes associated with aging [98]. Dysphagia, dementia, poor oral hygiene, and multiple comorbidities are risk factors for aspiration pneumonia [163]. Aspiration precautions should be taken for high risk patients, especially for those with neurologic conditions such as dementia or Parkinson's disease [129].

Patient falls are another concern common to the geriatric population and they are associated with an increased risk of subsequent death [164, 165]. Falls result from susceptible individuals being in a hazardous environment. Age associated changes in posture and decreased muscle strength increase vulnerability [166]. Impairment of gait, balance, vision, cognition, and function are risk factors [166]. Another risk factor for elderly falls is lower urinary tract symptoms, especially nocturia and urge incontinence [167]. Use of anti-cholinergic medications also increases fall risk [168]. Patients with a history of falls are more likely to fall again [166]. A post fall anxiety syndrome may develop which results in self-imposed restriction in ambulation and activity [169]. Screening for fall risk and nursing assistance whenever getting out of bed are the cornerstones of prevention.

Discharge Planning

Discharge planning should begin prior to admission for all patients, but especially for geriatric patients. Early discharge planning also assists in obtainment of needed resources, such as acute rehabilitation facilities, which are commonly needed for elderly patients. Making these arrangements as soon as possible allows for an efficient hospital discharge and avoids delays to find placement. A discussion about advance directives and healthcare proxy should occur with all patients, regardless of age.

Information on co-morbidities, functional status, and nutritional state obtained during the preoperative assessment will be important to determine placement needs. Consideration of social support, such as marital status, living situation, and potential caregivers, must also be factored into disposition planning. A recent Cochrane review showed that individualized discharge planning reduced length of stay and risk of readmission for elderly patients [170].

Discharge planning should focus on patient participation and education [171]. Outpatient education prior to surgery is particularly beneficial to elderly patients, who may have difficulty remembering information when in pain and on pain medications [172].

Patients with urinary diversions should have early follow-up with a stoma care specialist to optimize care and improve quality of life [173]. Family members and care givers should be encouraged to attend because many patients do not care for their urostomy independently [174].

For many major surgeries, such as radical cystectomy, there has been a shift towards decreasing length of hospital stay but increasing utilization of subacute care facilities and home health services [175]. Geriatric patients are at an increased risk of need for healthcare services at discharge. For example, older age as well as, lower preoperative albumin, unmarried status, and co-morbidity are predictors of need for home health services after radical cystectomy [176]. While older age, poor preoperative exercise tolerance, and longer hospital stay are potential risk factors for facility placement after cystectomy [176].

Prior to the patient's discharge, adequate communication with their outpatient geriatrician or primary care provider is important to ensure an appropriate transition of care. During the first few weeks following transurethral resection of the prostate, it is common for patients to contact their primary care provider with treatment-related concerns [177]. Similarly, despite claiming to very satisfied with teaching and information provided at discharge, many men will still use community healthcare resources following prostatectomy [178]. For geriatric patients with multiple medications, transition from an inpatient to outpatient setting must be well coordinated with their outpatient provider to reduce risk for medication and laboratory monitoring error [179]. Geriatric patients, especially with multiple comorbidities, should be encouraged to follow-up with their primary provider to reduce the risk of readmission [180].

Conclusion

The elderly population in the United States continues to grow in size. Advances in surgery and anesthesia have allowed for elderly patients to undergo operations that would not have been possible only a few decades ago. Clearly, chronologic age should not be a contraindication for any surgery. Optimal perioperative care of elderly surgical patients begins with a comprehensive preoperative assessment. Perioperative management and discharge planning should be individualized to achieve the best possible outcomes for the patient.

References

1. Etzioni DA, Liu JH, Maggard MA, Ko CY. The aging population and its impact on the surgery workforce. Ann Surg. 2003;238:170–7.
2. Day JC. Population projections of the United States, by age, sex, race, and Hispanic origin: 1993 to 2050. US Bureau of the Census, Current Population Reports. 1993. p. 25–1104.
3. Schuckman AK, Stein JP, Skinner D. Surgical considerations for elderly urologic oncology patients. Urol Oncol. 2009;27:628–32.
4. Liu LL, Wiener-Kronish JP. Perioperative anesthesia issues in the elderly. Crit Care Clin. 2003;19:641–56.
5. Bettelli G. Preoperative evaluation in geriatric surgery: comorbidity, functional status and pharmacological history. Minerva Anestesiol. 2011;77:637–46.
6. Turrentine FE, Wang H, Simpson VB, Jones RS. Surgical risk factors, morbidity, and mortality in elderly patients. J Am Coll Surg. 2006;203:865–77.
7. Manku K, Bacchetti P, Leung JM. Prognostic significance of postoperative in-hospital complications in elderly patients I. Long-term survival. Anesth Analg. 2003;96:583–9.
8. Wilder RJ, Fishbein RH. The widening surgical frontier. Postgrad Med. 1961;29:548–51.
9. Hamel MB, Henderson WG, Khuri SF, Daley J. Surgical outcomes for patients aged 80 and older: morbidity and mortality from major noncardiac surgery. J Am Geriatr Soc. 2005;53:424–9.
10. Bentrem DJ, Cohen ME, Hynes DM, Ko CY, Bilimoria KY. Identification of specific quality improvement opportunities for the elderly undergoing gastrointestinal surgery. Arch Surg. 2009;144:1013–20.
11. Lubin M. Surgery in the elderly. In: Lubin M, editor. Medical management of the surgical patient. 4th ed. Cambridge: Cambridge University Press; 2006.
12. Brody JP, Persky VW. Epidemiology and demographics. In: Abrams WB, Berkow R, editors. The Merck manual of geriatrics. Rahway, NJ: Merck Sharp & Dohme; 1990.
13. Hennus PM, Kroeze SG, Bosch JL, Jans JJ. Impact of comorbidity on complications after nephrectomy: use of the Clavien Classification of Surgical Complications. BJU Int. 2012;110: 682-7.
14. Resorlu B, Diri A, Atmaca AF, et al. Can we avoid percutaneous nephrolithotomy in high-risk elderly patients using the Charlson comorbidity index? Urology. 2011;79(5):1042–7.
15. Matin SF, Abreu S, Ramani A, et al. Evaluation of age and comorbidity as risk factors after laparoscopic urological surgery. J Urol. 2003;170:1115–20.
16. Guzzo TJ, Drach GW. Major urologic problems in geriatrics: assessment and management. Med Clin North Am. 2011;95:253–64.
17. Barnett SR. Polypharmacy and perioperative medications in the elderly. Anesthesiol Clin. 2009;27:377–89.
18. Karl A, Rittler P, Buchner A, et al. Prospective assessment of malnutrition in urologic patients. Urology. 2009;73:1072–6.
19. Gregg JR, Cookson MS, Phillips S, et al. Effect of preoperative nutritional deficiency on mortality after radical cystectomy for bladder cancer. J Urol. 2011;185:90–6.
20. Rosenthal RA, Kavic SM. Assessment and management of the geriatric patient. Crit Care Med. 2004;32:S92–105.
21. Howard L, Ashley C. Nutrition in the perioperative patient. Annu Rev Nutr. 2003;23: 263–82.
22. Karl A, Staehler M, Bauer R, et al. Malnutrition and clinical outcome in urological patients. Eur J Med Res. 2011;16:469–72.
23. Morgan TM, Keegan KA, Barocas DA, et al. Predicting the probability of 90-day survival of elderly patients with bladder cancer treated with radical cystectomy. J Urol. 2011;186:829–34.
24. Gibbs J, Cull W, Henderson W, Daley J, Hur K, Khuri SF. Preoperative serum albumin level as a predictor of operative mortality and morbidity: results from the National VA Surgical Risk Study. Arch Surg. 1999;134:36–42.

25. Moskovitz DN, Kim YI. Does perioperative immunonutrition reduce postoperative complications in patients with gastrointestinal cancer undergoing operations? Nutr Rev. 2004;62:443–7.
26. Mullen JT, Davenport DL, Hutter MM, et al. Impact of body mass index on perioperative outcomes in patients undergoing major intra-abdominal cancer surgery. Ann Surg Oncol. 2008;15:2164–72.
27. McClave SA, Snider HL, Spain DA. Preoperative issues in clinical nutrition. Chest. 1999;115:64S–70S.
28. Li P, Yin YL, Li D, Kim SW, Wu G. Amino acids and immune function. Br J Nutr. 2007;98:237–52.
29. Chandra RK. Nutrition and immunology: from the clinic to cellular biology and back again. Proc Nutr Soc. 1999;58:681–3.
30. Lesourd BM. Nutrition and immunity in the elderly: modification of immune responses with nutritional treatments. Am J Clin Nutr. 1997;66:478S–84S.
31. Mohler JL, Flanigan RC. The effect of nutritional status and support on morbidity and mortality of bladder cancer patients treated by radical cystectomy. J Urol. 1987;137:404–7.
32. Barrass BJ, Thurairaja R, Collins JW, Gillatt D, Persad RA. Optimal nutrition should improve the outcome and costs of radical cystectomy. Urol Int. 2006;77:139–42.
33. Maffezzini M, Campodonico F, Canepa G, Gerbi G, Parodi D. Current perioperative management of radical cystectomy with intestinal urinary reconstruction for muscle-invasive bladder cancer and reduction of the incidence of postoperative ileus. Surg Oncol. 2008;17:41–8.
34. Pruthi RS, Chun J, Richman M. Reducing time to oral diet and hospital discharge in patients undergoing radical cystectomy using a perioperative care plan. Urology. 2003;62:661–5; discussion 65–6.
35. Baldwin C, Spiro A, Ahern R, Emery PW. Oral nutritional interventions in malnourished patients with cancer: a systematic review and meta-analysis. J Natl Cancer Inst. 2012; 104:371–85.
36. Braga M, Gianotti L, Nespoli L, Radaelli G, Di Carlo V. Nutritional approach in malnourished surgical patients: a prospective randomized study. Arch Surg. 2002;137:174–80.
37. Visser M. Towards a definition of sarcopenia–results from epidemiologic studies. J Nutr Health Aging. 2009;13:713–6.
38. Newman AB, Kupelian V, Visser M, et al. Sarcopenia: alternative definitions and associations with lower extremity function. J Am Geriatr Soc. 2003;51:1602–9.
39. Tzankoff SP, Norris AH. Longitudinal changes in basal metabolism in man. J Appl Physiol. 1978;45:536–9.
40. Visser M, van Venrooij LM, Vulperhorst L, et al. Sarcopenic obesity is associated with adverse clinical outcome after cardiac surgery. Nutr Metab Cardiovasc Dis. 2012 Mar 6. [Epub ahead of print].
41. Prado CM, Lieffers JR, McCargar LJ, et al. Prevalence and clinical implications of sarcopenic obesity in patients with solid tumours of the respiratory and gastrointestinal tracts: a population-based study. Lancet Oncol. 2008;9:629–35.
42. Goodpaster BH, Park SW, Harris TB, et al. The loss of skeletal muscle strength, mass, and quality in older adults: the health, aging and body composition study. J Gerontol A Biol Sci Med Sci. 2006;61:1059–64.
43. Newman AB, Kupelian V, Visser M, et al. Strength, but not muscle mass, is associated with mortality in the health, aging and body composition study cohort. J Gerontol A Biol Sci Med Sci. 2006;61:72–7.
44. Studenski S, Perera S, Patel K, et al. Gait speed and survival in older adults. JAMA. 2011;305:50–8.
45. Cohn SH, Vartsky D, Yasumura S, et al. Compartmental body composition based on total-body nitrogen, potassium, and calcium. Am J Physiol. 1980;239:E524–30.
46. Zamboni M, Mazzali G, Fantin F, Rossi A, Di Francesco V. Sarcopenic obesity: a new category of obesity in the elderly. Nutr Metab Cardiovasc Dis. 2008;18:88–95.

47. Jensen GL, Hsiao PY. Obesity in older adults: relationship to functional limitation. Curr Opin Clin Nutr Metab Care. 2010;13:46–51.
48. Bamgbade OA, Rutter TW, Nafiu OO, Dorje P. Postoperative complications in obese and nonobese patients. World J Surg. 2007;31:556–60; discussion 61.
49. Manton KG. A longitudinal study of functional change and mortality in the United States. J Gerontol. 1988;43:S153–61.
50. Seymour DG, Pringle R. Post-operative complications in the elderly surgical patient. Gerontology. 1983;29:262–70.
51. Stefan M, Iglesia Lino L, Fernandez G. Medical consultation and best practices for preoperative evaluation of elderly patients. Hosp Pract (Minneap). 2011;39:41–51.
52. Ostir GV, Berges I, Kuo YF, Goodwin JS, Ottenbacher KJ, Guralnik JM. Assessing gait speed in acutely ill older patients admitted to an acute care for elders hospital unit. Arch Intern Med. 2012;172:353–8.
53. Kristjansson SR, Nesbakken A, Jordhoy MS, et al. Comprehensive geriatric assessment can predict complications in elderly patients after elective surgery for colorectal cancer: a prospective observational cohort study. Crit Rev Oncol Hematol. 2010;76:208–17.
54. Mohile SG, Bylow K, Dale W, et al. A pilot study of the vulnerable elders survey-13 compared with the comprehensive geriatric assessment for identifying disability in older patients with prostate cancer who receive androgen ablation. Cancer. 2007;109:802–10.
55. Pasetto LM, Lise M, Monfardini S. Preoperative assessment of elderly cancer patients. Crit Rev Oncol Hematol. 2007;64:10–8.
56. Froehner M, Hentschel C, Koch R, Litz RJ, Hakenberg OW, Wirth MP. Which comorbidity classification best fits elderly candidates for radical prostatectomy? Urol Oncol. 2011 Apr 15. [Epub ahead of print].
57. Glance LG, Lustik SJ, Hannan EL, et al. The surgical mortality probability model: derivation and validation of a simple risk prediction rule for noncardiac surgery. Ann Surg. 2012;255:696–702.
58. Froehner M, Koch R, Litz RJ, et al. Detailed analysis of Charlson comorbidity score as predictor of mortality after radical prostatectomy. Urology. 2008;72:1252–7.
59. Guzzo TJ, Dluzniewski P, Orosco R, Platz EA, Partin AW, Han M. Prediction of mortality after radical prostatectomy by Charlson comorbidity index. Urology. 2010;76:553–7.
60. Salvi F, Miller MD, Grilli A, et al. A manual of guidelines to score the modified cumulative illness rating scale and its validation in acute hospitalized elderly patients. J Am Geriatr Soc. 2008;56:926–31.
61. Fortin M, Steenbakkers K, Hudon C, Poitras ME, Almirall J, van den Akker M. The electronic Cumulative Illness Rating Scale: a reliable and valid tool to assess multi-morbidity in primary care. J Eval Clin Pract. 2011;17:1089–93.
62. Audisio RA, Pope D, Ramesh HS, et al. Shall we operate? Preoperative assessment in elderly cancer patients (PACE) can help. A SIOG surgical task force prospective study. Crit Rev Oncol Hematol. 2008;65:156–63.
63. Makary MA, Segev DL, Pronovost PJ, et al. Frailty as a predictor of surgical outcomes in older patients. J Am Coll Surg. 2010;210:901–8.
64. Chikwe J, Adams DH. Frailty: the missing element in predicting operative mortality. Semin Thorac Cardiovasc Surg. 2010;22:109–10.
65. Tan KY, Kawamura YJ, Tokomitsu A, Tang T. Assessment for frailty is useful for predicting morbidity in elderly patients undergoing colorectal cancer resection whose comorbidities are already optimized. Am J Surg. 2012;204: 139-43.
66. Woolger JM. Preoperative testing and medication management. Clin Geriatr Med. 2008;24:573–83, vii.
67. Marcello PW, Roberts PL. "Routine" preoperative studies. Which studies in which patients? Surg Clin North Am. 1996;76:11–23.
68. Velanovich V. Preoperative laboratory evaluation. J Am Coll Surg. 1996;183:79–87.
69. Fischer SP. Cost-effective preoperative evaluation and testing. Chest. 1999;115:96S–100S.

70. Johnstone RE, Martinec CL. Costs of anesthesia. Anesth Analg. 1993;76:840–8.
71. Dzankic S, Pastor D, Gonzalez C, Leung JM. The prevalence and predictive value of abnormal preoperative laboratory tests in elderly surgical patients. Anesth Analg. 2001;93:301–8.
72. Reilly DF, McNeely MJ, Doerner D, et al. Self-reported exercise tolerance and the risk of serious perioperative complications. Arch Intern Med. 1999;159:2185–92.
73. Gerson MC, Hurst JM, Hertzberg VS, et al. Cardiac prognosis in noncardiac geriatric surgery. Ann Intern Med. 1985;103:832–7.
74. Gerson MC, Hurst JM, Hertzberg VS, Baughman R, Rouan GW, Ellis K. Prediction of cardiac and pulmonary complications related to elective abdominal and noncardiac thoracic surgery in geriatric patients. Am J Med. 1990;88:101–7.
75. Michota FA, Frost SD. Perioperative management of the hospitalized patient. Med Clin North Am. 2002;86:731–48.
76. Goldman L, Caldera DL, Nussbaum SR, et al. Multifactorial index of cardiac risk in noncardiac surgical procedures. N Engl J Med. 1977;297:845–50.
77. Detsky AS, Abrams HB, Forbath N, Scott JG, Hilliard JR. Cardiac assessment for patients undergoing noncardiac surgery. A multifactorial clinical risk index. Arch Intern Med. 1986;146:2131–4.
78. Lee TH, Marcantonio ER, Mangione CM, et al. Derivation and prospective validation of a simple index for prediction of cardiac risk of major noncardiac surgery. Circulation. 1999;100:1043–9.
79. Boersma E, Kertai MD, Schouten O, et al. Perioperative cardiovascular mortality in noncardiac surgery: validation of the Lee cardiac risk index. Am J Med. 2005;118:1134–41.
80. Sox Jr HC, Garber AM, Littenberg B. The resting electrocardiogram as a screening test. A clinical analysis. Ann Intern Med. 1989;111:489–502.
81. Seymour DG, Pringle R, MacLennan WJ. The role of the routine pre-operative electrocardiogram in the elderly surgical patient. Age Ageing. 1983;12:97–104.
82. Zaugg M, Lucchinetti E. Respiratory function in the elderly. Anesthesiol Clin North Am. 2000;18:47–58, vi.
83. Warner MA, Offord KP, Warner ME, Lennon RL, Conover MA, Jansson-Schumacher U. Role of preoperative cessation of smoking and other factors in postoperative pulmonary complications: a blinded prospective study of coronary artery bypass patients. Mayo Clin Proc. 1989;64:609–16.
84. Fleshner N, Garland J, Moadel A, et al. Influence of smoking status on the disease-related outcomes of patients with tobacco-associated superficial transitional cell carcinoma of the bladder. Cancer. 1999;86:2337–45.
85. Chen CH, Shun CT, Huang KH, et al. Stopping smoking might reduce tumour recurrence in nonmuscle-invasive bladder cancer. BJU Int. 2007;100:281–6; discussion 86.
86. Brennan P, Bogillot O, Cordier S, et al. Cigarette smoking and bladder cancer in men: a pooled analysis of 11 case–control studies. Int J Cancer. 2000;86:289–94.
87. Guzzo TJ, Hockenberry MS, Mucksavage P, Bivalacqua TJ, Schoenberg MP. Smoking knowledge assessment and cessation trends in patients with bladder cancer presenting to a tertiary referral center. Urology. 2012;79:166–71.
88. Bjurlin MA, Goble SM, Hollowell CM. Smoking cessation assistance for patients with bladder cancer: a national survey of American urologists. J Urol. 2010;184:1901–6.
89. Jugdutt BI. Heart failure in the elderly: advances and challenges. Expert Rev Cardiovasc Ther. 2010;8:695–715.
90. Priebe HJ. The aged cardiovascular risk patient. Br J Anaesth. 2000;85:763–78.
91. Deiner S, Silverstein JH. Anesthesia for geriatric patients. Minerva Anestesiol. 2011;77:180–9.
92. Rooke GA. Autonomic and cardiovascular function in the geriatric patient. Anesthesiol Clin North America. 2000;18:31–46, v–vi.
93. Sanders D, Dudley M, Groban L. Diastolic dysfunction, cardiovascular aging, and the anesthesiologist. Anesthesiol Clin. 2009;27:497–517.

94. Brown WW, Davis BB, Spry LA, Wongsurawat N, Malone JD, Domoto DT. Aging and the kidney. Arch Intern Med. 1986;146:1790–6.
95. Epstein CD, Peerless JR. Weaning readiness and fluid balance in older critically ill surgical patients. Am J Crit Care. 2006;15:54–64.
96. Cohn SH, Gartenhaus W, Sawitsky A, et al. Compartmental body composition of cancer patients by measurement of total body nitrogen, potassium, and water. Metabolism. 1981;30:222–9.
97. McLachlan AJ, Pont LG. Drug metabolism in older people–a key consideration in achieving optimal outcomes with medicines. J Gerontol A Biol Sci Med Sci. 2012;67:175–80.
98. Erskine RJ, Murphy PJ, Langton JA, Smith G. Effect of age on the sensitivity of upper airway reflexes. Br J Anaesth. 1993;70:574–5.
99. Akhavan A, Gainsburg DM, Stock JA. Complications associated with patient positioning in urologic surgery. Urology. 2010;76:1309–16.
100. Schultz A. Predicting and preventing pressure ulcers in surgical patients. AORN J. 2005;81: 986–1006; quiz 09–12.
101. Warner MA. Perioperative neuropathies. Mayo Clin Proc. 1998;73:567–74.
102. Felson DT, Naimark A, Anderson J, Kazis L, Castelli W, Meenan RF. The prevalence of knee osteoarthritis in the elderly. The Framingham Osteoarthritis Study. Arthritis Rheum. 1987;30:914–8.
103. Molloy BL. Implications for postoperative visual loss: steep trendelenburg position and effects on intraocular pressure. AANA J. 2011;79:115–21.
104. Gainsburg DM. Anesthetic concerns for robotic-assisted laparoscopic radical prostatectomy. Minerva Anestesiol. 2012;78(5):596–604.
105. Gill IS, Kavoussi LR, Lane BR, et al. Comparison of 1,800 laparoscopic and open partial nephrectomies for single renal tumors. J Urol. 2007;178:41–6.
106. Gong EM, Orvieto MA, Zorn KC, Lucioni A, Steinberg GD, Shalhav AL. Comparison of laparoscopic and open partial nephrectomy in clinical T1a renal tumors. J Endourol. 2008;22:953–7.
107. Lotan Y, Cadeddu JA. A cost comparison of nephron-sparing surgical techniques for renal tumour. BJU Int. 2005;95:1039–42.
108. Marcantonio ER, Goldman L, Orav EJ, Cook EF, Lee TH. The association of intraoperative factors with the development of postoperative delirium. Am J Med. 1998;105:380–4.
109. Ramani AP, Desai MM, Steinberg AP, et al. Complications of laparoscopic partial nephrectomy in 200 cases. J Urol. 2005;173:42–7.
110. Ng CK, Kauffman EC, Lee MM, et al. A comparison of postoperative complications in open versus robotic cystectomy. Eur Urol. 2010;57:274–81.
111. Eagle KA, Rihal CS, Mickel MC, Holmes DR, Foster ED, Gersh BJ. Cardiac risk of noncardiac surgery: influence of coronary disease and type of surgery in 3368 operations. CASS Investigators and University of Michigan Heart Care Program. Coronary Artery Surgery Study. Circulation. 1997;96:1882–7.
112. Dunkelgrun M, Boersma E, Schouten O, et al. Bisoprolol and fluvastatin for the reduction of perioperative cardiac mortality and myocardial infarction in intermediate-risk patients undergoing noncardiovascular surgery: a randomized controlled trial (DECREASE-IV). Ann Surg. 2009;249:921–6.
113. Mangano DT, Wong MG, London MJ, Tubau JF, Rapp JA. Perioperative myocardial ischemia in patients undergoing noncardiac surgery–II: incidence and severity during the 1st week after surgery. The Study of Perioperative Ischemia (SPI) Research Group. J Am Coll Cardiol. 1991;17:851–7.
114. Mangano DT, Hollenberg M, Fegert G, et al. Perioperative myocardial ischemia in patients undergoing noncardiac surgery–I: incidence and severity during the 4 day perioperative period. The Study of Perioperative Ischemia (SPI) Research Group. J Am Coll Cardiol. 1991;17:843–50.
115. Poldermans D, Boersma E, Bax JJ, et al. The effect of bisoprolol on perioperative mortality and myocardial infarction in high-risk patients undergoing vascular surgery. Dutch

Echocardiographic Cardiac Risk Evaluation Applying Stress Echocardiography Study Group. N Engl J Med. 1999;341:1789–94.

116. Devereaux PJ, Yang H, Yusuf S, et al. Effects of extended-release metoprolol succinate in patients undergoing non-cardiac surgery (POISE trial): a randomised controlled trial. Lancet. 2008;371:1839–47.

117. Davignon J. Beneficial cardiovascular pleiotropic effects of statins. Circulation. 2004;109:III39–43.

118. Hindler K, Shaw AD, Samuels J, Fulton S, Collard CD, Riedel B. Improved postoperative outcomes associated with preoperative statin therapy. Anesthesiology. 2006;105:1260–72; quiz 89–90.

119. Spencer FA, Fonarow GC, Frederick PD, et al. Early withdrawal of statin therapy in patients with non-ST-segment elevation myocardial infarction: national registry of myocardial infarction. Arch Intern Med. 2004;164:2162–8.

120. Singh PP, Srinivasa S, Lemanu DP, Maccormick AD, Hill AG. Statins in abdominal surgery: a systematic review. J Am Coll Surg. 2012;214:356–66.

121. Patrono C, Garcia Rodriguez LA, Landolfi R, Baigent C. Low-dose aspirin for the prevention of atherothrombosis. N Engl J Med. 2005;353:2373–83.

122. Vinik R, Yarbrough P. Perioperative management of cardiac issues in the patient undergoing genitourinary surgery. AUA update series. 2010. Volume 29, Lesson 1.

123. Noordzij PG, Boersma E, Schreiner F, et al. Increased preoperative glucose levels are associated with perioperative mortality in patients undergoing noncardiac, nonvascular surgery. Eur J Endocrinol. 2007;156:137–42.

124. Maynard G, O'Malley CW, Kirsh SR. Perioperative care of the geriatric patient with diabetes or hyperglycemia. Clin Geriatr Med. 2008;24:649–65, viii.

125. Hong M, Yoon H. [Influence of pre-operative fasting time on blood glucose in older patients]. J Korean Acad Nurs. 2011;41:157–64.

126. Kratzing C. Pre-operative nutrition and carbohydrate loading. Proc Nutr Soc. 2011; 70:311–5.

127. Torossian A. Thermal management during anaesthesia and thermoregulation standards for the prevention of inadvertent perioperative hypothermia. Best Pract Res Clin Anaesthesiol. 2008;22:659–68.

128. Kurz A. Thermal care in the perioperative period. Best Pract Res Clin Anaesthesiol. 2008; 22:39–62.

129. Sieber FE, Barnett SR. Preventing postoperative complications in the elderly. Anesthesiol Clin. 2011;29:83–97.

130. Gawande AA, Regenbogen SE. Critical need for objective assessment of postsurgical patients. Anesthesiology. 2011;114:1269–70.

131. Awad IT, Chung F. Factors affecting recovery and discharge following ambulatory surgery. Can J Anaesth. 2006;53:858–72.

132. Fredman B, Sheffer O, Zohar E, et al. Fast-track eligibility of geriatric patients undergoing short urologic surgery procedures. Anesth Analg. 2002;94:560–4.

133. Chung F. Discharge criteria–a new trend. Can J Anaesth. 1995;42:1056–8.

134. Regenbogen SE, Ehrenfeld JM, Lipsitz SR, Greenberg CC, Hutter MM, Gawande AA. Utility of the surgical apgar score: validation in 4119 patients. Arch Surg. 2009;144:30–6; discussion 37.

135. Pisani MA. Considerations in caring for the critically ill older patient. J Intensive Care Med. 2009;24:83–95.

136. Marik PE. Management of the critically ill geriatric patient. Crit Care Med. 2006; 34:S176–82.

137. Prasad SM, Ferreria M, Berry AM, et al. Surgical apgar outcome score: perioperative risk assessment for radical cystectomy. J Urol. 2009;181:1046–52; discussion 52–3.

138. Kwok AC, Lipsitz SR, Bader AM, Gawande AA. Are targeted preoperative risk prediction tools more powerful? A test of models for emergency colon surgery in the very elderly. J Am Coll Surg. 2011;213:220–5.

139. Kaufman MR, Baumgartner RG, Anderson LW, et al. The evidence-based pathway for peri-operative management of open and robotically assisted laparoscopic radical prostatectomy. BJU Int. 2007;99:1103–8.
140. Chang SS, Cole E, Smith Jr JA, Baumgartner R, Wells N, Cookson MS. Safely reducing length of stay after open radical retropubic prostatectomy under the guidance of a clinical care pathway. Cancer. 2005;104:747–51.
141. Koch MO, Smith Jr JA. Influence of patient age and co-morbidity on outcome of a collaborative care pathway after radical prostatectomy and cystoprostatectomy. J Urol. 1996; 155:1681–4.
142. Stagg P, Grice T. Nasogastric medication for perioperative Parkinson's rigidity during anaesthesia emergence. Anaesth Intensive Care. 2011;39:1128–30.
143. Ong J, Miller PS, Appleby R, Allegretto R, Gawlinski A. Effect of a preoperative instructional digital video disc on patient knowledge and preparedness for engaging in postoperative care activities. Nurs Clin North Am. 2009;44:103–15, xii.
144. Browning L, Denehy L, Scholes RL. The quantity of early upright mobilisation performed following upper abdominal surgery is low: an observational study. Aust J Physiother. 2007;53:47–52.
145. Sindell S, Causey MW, Bradley T, Poss M, Moonka R, Thirlby R. Expediting return of bowel function after colorectal surgery. Am J Surg. 2012;203(5):644–8.
146. Killewich LA. Strategies to minimize postoperative deconditioning in elderly surgical patients. J Am Coll Surg. 2006;203:735–45.
147. Gould MK, Garcia DA, Wren SM, et al. Prevention of VTE in nonorthopedic surgical patients: Antithrombotic Therapy and Prevention of Thrombosis, 9th ed: American College of Chest Physicians Evidence-Based Clinical Practice Guidelines. Chest. 2012;141: e227S–77S.
148. Stratton MA, Anderson FA, Bussey HI, et al. Prevention of venous thromboembolism: adherence to the 1995 American College of Chest Physicians consensus guidelines for surgical patients. Arch Intern Med. 2000;160:334–40.
149. Forrest JB, Clemens JQ, Finamore P, et al. AUA Best Practice Statement for the prevention of deep vein thrombosis in patients undergoing urologic surgery. J Urol. 2009;181:1170–7.
150. Warren J, Bhalla V, Cresci G. Postoperative diet advancement: surgical dogma vs evidence-based medicine. Nutr Clin Pract. 2011;26:115–25.
151. Luckey AE, Parsa CJ. Fluid and electrolytes in the aged. Arch Surg. 2003;138:1055–60.
152. Brady M, Kinn S, Stuart P. Preoperative fasting for adults to prevent perioperative complications. Cochrane Database Syst Rev. 2003:CD004423.
153. Washington LL, Gibson SJ, Helme RD. Age-related differences in the endogenous analgesic response to repeated cold water immersion in human volunteers. Pain. 2000;89:89–96.
154. Lynch EP, Lazor MA, Gellis JE, Orav J, Goldman L, Marcantonio ER. The impact of postoperative pain on the development of postoperative delirium. Anesth Analg. 1998;86:781–5.
155. Mercadante S. Intravenous patient-controlled analgesia and management of pain in postsurgical elderly with cancer. Surg Oncol. 2010;19:173–7.
156. Mann C, Pouzeratte Y, Boccara G, et al. Comparison of intravenous or epidural patient-controlled analgesia in the elderly after major abdominal surgery. Anesthesiology. 2000;92:433–41.
157. Aubrun F, Marmion F. The elderly patient and postoperative pain treatment. Best Pract Res Clin Anaesthesiol. 2007;21:109–27.
158. Parikh SS, Chung F. Postoperative delirium in the elderly. Anesth Analg. 1995;80:1223–32.
159. Cole MG, Primeau FJ. Prognosis of delirium in elderly hospital patients. CMAJ. 1993;149:41–6.
160. Inouye SK. Delirium in older persons. N Engl J Med. 2006;354:1157–65.
161. Franco K, Litaker D, Locala J, Bronson D. The cost of delirium in the surgical patient. Psychosomatics. 2001;42:68–73.
162. Marcantonio ER, Flacker JM, Wright RJ, Resnick NM. Reducing delirium after hip fracture: a randomized trial. J Am Geriatr Soc. 2001;49:516–22.

163. Sue Eisenstadt E. Dysphagia and aspiration pneumonia in older adults. J Am Acad Nurse Pract. 2010;22:17–22.
164. Sylliaas H, Idland G, Sandvik L, Forsen L, Bergland A. Does mortality of the aged increase with the number of falls? Results from a nine-year follow-up study. Eur J Epidemiol. 2009;24:351–5.
165. Alamgir H, Muazzam S, Nasrullah M. Unintentional falls mortality among elderly in the United States: time for action. Injury. 2012 Jan 18. [Epub ahead of print].
166. Bradley SM. Falls in older adults. Mt Sinai J Med. 2011;78:590–5.
167. Parsons JK, Mougey J, Lambert L, et al. Lower urinary tract symptoms increase the risk of falls in older men. BJU Int. 2009;104:63–8.
168. Berdot S, Bertrand M, Dartigues JF, et al. Inappropriate medication use and risk of falls–a prospective study in a large community-dwelling elderly cohort. BMC Geriatr. 2009;9:30.
169. Rubenstein LZ, Josephson KR. Falls and their prevention in elderly people: what does the evidence show? Med Clin North Am. 2006;90:807–24.
170. Shepperd S, McClaran J, Phillips CO, et al. Discharge planning from hospital to home. Cochrane Database Syst Rev. 2010:CD000313.
171. Carroll A, Dowling M. Discharge planning: communication, education and patient participation. Br J Nurs. 2007;16:882–6.
172. Merriman ML. Pre-hospital discharge planning: empowering elderly patients through choice. Crit Care Nurs Q. 2008;31:52–8.
173. O'Connor G. Discharge planning in rehabilitation following surgery for a stoma. Br J Nurs. 2003;12:800–7.
174. Tal R, Cohen MM, Yossepowitch O, et al. An ileal conduit-who takes care of the stoma? J Urol. 2012;187:1707–12.
175. Taub DA, Dunn RL, Miller DC, Wei JT, Hollenbeck BK. Discharge practice patterns following cystectomy for bladder cancer: evidence for the shifting of the burden of care. J Urol. 2006;176:2612–7; discussion 17–8.
176. Aghazadeh MA, Barocas DA, Salem S, et al. Determining factors for hospital discharge status after radical cystectomy in a large contemporary cohort. J Urol. 2011;185:85–9.
177. Mogensen K, Jacobsen JD. The load on family and primary healthcare in the first six weeks after transurethral resection of the prostate. Scand J Urol Nephrol. 2008;42:132–6.
178. Davison BJ, Moore KN, MacMillan H, Bisaillon A, Wiens K. Patient evaluation of a discharge program following a radical prostatectomy. Urol Nurs. 2004;24:483–9.
179. Moore C, Wisnivesky J, Williams S, McGinn T. Medical errors related to discontinuity of care from an inpatient to an outpatient setting. J Gen Intern Med. 2003;18:646–51.
180. Misky GJ, Wald HL, Coleman EA. Post-hospitalization transitions: examining the effects of timing of primary care provider follow-up. J Hosp Med. 2010;5:392–7.

Chapter 6
Complications Particular to the Elderly

Andrew M. Harris and Thomas J. Guzzo

Introduction

As medicine has continued to make advances and life expectancy has increased, the patients presenting for surgical intervention have continued to get older. People over the age of 85 are the fastest growing age class in our society today [1]. Those patients 65 years old and older are expected to be 20% of our population by 2025 [2]. More than half of these individuals will undergo major surgery, most after the age of 50 [2]. These patients are more likely to have cardiopulmonary disease, diabetes, and other health problems and are more likely to have elective surgery canceled [1, 2]. This patient population is more likely to present with advanced disease and require emergent surgery and also has higher mortality when compared to younger patients [1, 2].

Operating on the elderly isn't without increased risk. The 30 day mortality increases by nearly 10% for every year over age 70 [3]. Those patients with an increased ASA (American Society of Anesthesiologists') score and decreased albumin are at increased risk of postoperative complications and mortality [3]. The National Surgical Quality Improvement Program showed the 30-day mortality for patients over the age of 80 was 8% and the surgical complication rate was 20% [3]. Another study of patients over 70 years of age undergoing surgery found a 20% complication rate within 5 days and a 6% mortality rate within the first 30 days. This same study also found many patients had more than one complication for an average of 31 complications per 100 patients [3]. The incidence of these

A.M. Harris
Department of Urology, Hospital of the University of Pennsylvania,
Philadelphia, PA 19404, USA
e-mail: amharr2@gmail.com

T.J. Guzzo (✉)
Department of Surgery, Division or Urology, Perelman Center for Advanced Medicine,
Hospital of the University of Pennsylvania, Philadelphia, PA 19404, USA
e-mail: thomas.guzzo@uphs.upenn.edu

T.J. Guzzo et al. (eds.), *Primer of Geriatric Urology*, DOI 10.1007/978-1-4614-4773-3_6,   65
© Springer Science+Business Media New York 2013

complications affects morbidity and mortality. The primary goal should be to prevent complications rather than treat them. However, when a complication does occur, it must be recognized and dealt with expeditiously and vigilantly to prevent further harm to the patient, particularly in the elderly population who often have less functional reserve. The most common and severe complications to affect the elderly population are deep vein thromboembolism, functional loss, immobility, delirium, postoperative cognitive dysfunction, urinary tract infection, falls, and a newer concept known as frailty.

Deep Vein Thrombosis

While the exact etiology is unclear, elderly patients are at increased risk of pulmonary venous thromboembolism when compared to younger patients and experience greater morbidity and mortality as well [4]. To understand why this population is at increased risk, it is important to remember the main factors contributing to venous thromboembolism as indicated in Virchow's triad: venous stasis, hypercoagulability, and intimal injury [4]. According to recent studies, immobility is the most prevalent risk factor for pulmonary embolism [4]. Elderly patients, especially those with frailty (see below), are more likely to be immobile in the postoperative period, thus putting them at higher risk for such events. Patients with heart failure are also at increased risk for thromboembolism [4] and elderly patients are more likely to have heart failure [5]. Anesthesia leads to venous dilation and, therefore, venous stasis, thus making it a risk factor for thromboembolism [4].

Elderly patients also have less fibrinolytic activity in leg veins than in arm veins, thus making deep venous thromboembolism more likely [4]. This population also has higher fibrinogen levels and higher procoagulant factors when compared to a younger population [4]. All of these factors put the elderly patient at increased risk for venous thromboembolism.

The most significant complication of DVT is pulmonary embolism (PE), which occurs more frequently in the elderly population [4]. The incidence of PE is 1.8% in those aged 65–69, but increases to 3.1% in the 85–89-year-old population. When compared to age 20, an 80-year-old is 200 times more likely to have a PE [4]. Not only is PE more prevalent among the elderly population, this diagnosis also carries more morbidity and mortality as well. When compared with the general population, the elderly are 6 times more likely to die of a pulmonary embolism. The clinician must be continually keeping this diagnosis in the forefront of the mind in postoperative patients. Those patients experiencing dyspnea, tachycardia, tachypnea, and chest pain must be evaluated immediately to rule out an underlying PE.

Duplex ultrasound is the most commonly used study to evaluate for DVT; however, this study is most accurate when the patient has symptoms of lower extremity DVT. In the absence of symptoms, duplex ultrasonagraphy remains a very specific test. MRI with gadolinium is both sensitive and specific for DVT, but can be more difficult and expensive to obtain than a venous doppler [4]. Contrast venography is not used as often, but does remain the gold standard. The best treatment for DVT is prevention. DVT prophylaxis with low dose heparin or low molecular weight heparin are viable options [4].

Functional Loss/Immobility

The elderly patient faces significant barriers to postoperative mobility including increased incidence of arthritis, musculoskeletal problems, and quicker debilitation when compared to younger patients [2]. Prolonged bed rest in this population leads to significant pathophysiological complications in multiple organ systems [2]. The skin can be extremely affected by immobility in the form of pressure ulcers, which are associated with increased mortality [2]. Osteoporosis, by way of bone resorption, occurs at a faster rate in immobilized patients and increases fracture risk [2]. Immobility also leads to increased risk deep venous thromboembolism, pneumonia, aspiration, and atelectasis [2].

Immobility can lead to alterations in cardiac function manifested as hypotension and stroke [2]. The gastrointestinal system is also significantly affected by immobility, leading to decreased appetite and dehydration which can further exacerbate constipation and fecal impaction [2]. Immobility also affects cognition by leading to depression, altered sensorium, and loneliness [2]. Many of these complications are prevented by early mobilization and the work of a mulitfactorial team including nurses, physical therapists, family members, occupational therapists, physicians, and the patient's own cooperation [2].

Mental Disorders Associated with Aging

Delirium

Postoperative delirium, defined as incoherent speech, altered orientation, attention, emotional lability, and memory lapse for a short time period, accounts for longer hospital stays, increased cost, increased morbidity, mortality, and delayed functional recovery [1, 2, 6, 7]. This post operative complication costs over $4 billion per year [6]. Twenty percent of elderly surgical patients may experience postoperative delirium [2]. Delirium, which is usually reversible, tends to affect this patient population more in the evening hours and after postoperative day 1, peaking between postoperative days 2–7 [1, 6].

There are a multitude of risk factors for postoperative delirium, including age, preoperative cognitive function, ASA >II, medication interactions, withdrawal from medications being held in the postoperative period, alcohol withdrawal, insomnia, depression, dementia, anxiety, deficiencies in vision or hearing, and physical impairment [1, 2, 6].

There seems to be operation specific factors also contributing to postoperative delirium. The degree of operative stress is directly proportional to the risk of postoperative delirium, such that high stress procedures such as vascular surgery have a delirium risk of 36% but low stress procedures, such as cataract surgery, have a delirium risk of 4% [7].

Intraoperative events which may lead to delirium include those events leading to reduced oxygen delivery to the cerebral tissue such as: major blood loss, decreased hemoglobin, arterial hypoxemia, and hypotension [1, 2, 6]. The current working theory is that reduced oxygen delivery to the brain alters the neurotransmitter milieu in a detrimental fashion [6]. Surgery is known to cause alterations in stress hormone homeostasis which may also alter this milieu, possibly leading to delirium [6]. This condition may also increase the risk of more significant complications such as heart attack and pneumonia [2]. Interestingly, the type of anesthesia doesn't appear to have an effect on the incidence of postoperative delirium [1, 6].

Metabolic abnormalities during surgery can also play role in postoperative delirium [6]. Specifically, alterations in sodium, carbon dioxide levels, and overall fluid status, namely dehydration, are known to contribute to postoperative delirium. Pharmacokinetics vary widely among the elderly population and response as well as clearance of anesthetic is very difficult to predict. Perioperative anesthetic still present in the postoperative period likely contributes to postoperative delirium as well [6].

The clinician's focus should be on the prevention of rather than the treatment of postoperative delirium. Medical illnesses should be optimized prior to surgery and an up to date medication reconciliation should be done [6]. The patient should have adequate cerebral oxygen supply preoperatively and be adequately hydrated. An accurate drug and alcohol history should be obtained in order to identify and prevent postoperative withdrawal. Those patients with a history of alcohol abuse should be placed on thiamine to prevent Korsakoff's psychosis [6]. A proper postoperative pain control plan should be identified and carried out. The patient should be provided cerebral stimulation, optimal resting and sleeping conditions such as reduced noise levels, frequent orientation by the staff/family, easy access to visual aids like glasses, hearing aids, and early mobilization [6, 7]. These protocols may decrease postoperative delirium by 5% [7]. Clocks, calendars, windows, and appropriate daytime/nighttime lighting may also help keep the patient oriented [2]. The patient's electrolytes, oxygen levels, blood pressure, and fluid status should all be maintained appropriately in the perioperative and postoperative period [6, 7]. Tubes and drains should be managed vigilantly and removed as soon as possible as they have also been linked to postoperative delirium [7].

Once postoperative delirium occurs, it must be recognized in order to be treated appropriately. Up to half of delirium cases may be missed by the primary team [7]. Delirium must also be distinguished from postoperative cognitive dysfunction (POCD), which only affects memory, attention, and comprehension [7]. There are three main types of delirium: hyperactive, hypoactive, and mixed. Hypoactive delirium is the most common (71%), followed by mixed delirium (29%), while hyperactive is rare [7]. The hypoactive type of patient may be lethargic, unaware of his/her surroundings, and have decreased alertness [7]. The patient with hyperactive delirium has symptoms of irritability, agitation, restlessness, and may even be combative. The patient with mixed delirium has a combination of hypoactive and hyperactive delirium [7].

The Confusion Assessment Method (CAM-ICU) is a common test used to diagnose delirium in hospitalized patients (see Fig. 6.1) [6, 7]. This method provides a standardized system with high validity and reproducibility [6, 7]. CAM-ICU not

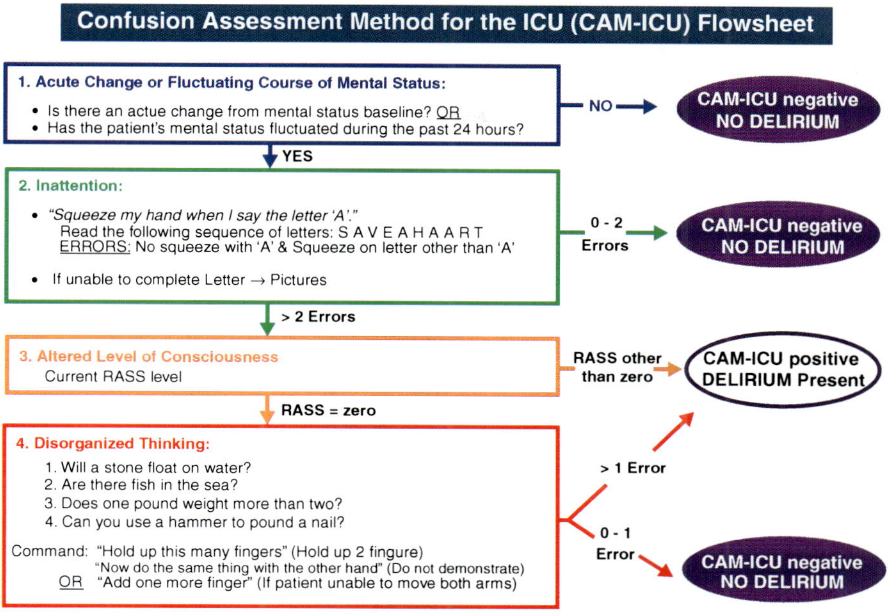

Confusion Assessment Method for the ICU (CAM-ICU) Flowsheet

1. Acute Change or Fluctuating Course of Mental Status:
- Is there an actue change from mental status baseline? OR
- Has the patient's mental status fluctuated during the past 24 hours?

NO → **CAM-ICU negative NO DELIRIUM**

↓ YES

2. Inattention:
- *"Squeeze my hand when I say the letter 'A'."*
  Read the following sequence of letters: S A V E A H A A R T
  ERRORS: No squeeze with 'A' & Squeeze on letter other than 'A'
- If unable to complete Letter → Pictures

0 - 2 Errors → **CAM-ICU negative NO DELIRIUM**

↓ > 2 Errors

3. Altered Level of Consciousness
Current RASS level

RASS other than zero → **CAM-ICU positive DELIRIUM Present**

↓ RASS = zero

4. Disorganized Thinking:
1. Will a stone float on water?
2. Are there fish in the sea?
3. Does one pound weight more than two?
4. Can you use a hammer to pound a nail?

Command: "Hold up this many fingers" (Hold up 2 fingure)
  "Now do the same thing with the other hand" (Do not demonstrate)
  OR   "Add one more finger" (If patient unable to move both arms)

> 1 Error → **CAM-ICU positive DELIRIUM Present**

0 - 1 Error → **CAM-ICU negative NO DELIRIUM**

Fig. 6.1 Confusion Assessment Method. Courtesy of Vanderbilt University. Available from: http://www.mc.vanderbilt.edu/icudelirium/docs/CAM_ICU_flowsheet.pdf

only examines mental status, thinking, and attention, but also level of consciousness. This assessment method can be used by both nurses and clinicians [7].

Treating postoperative delirium should focus on identifying risk factors, as well as underlying conditions, and treating them appropriately. A thorough history and physical should be done first [7]. Postoperative complications, including urinary tract infection, pneumonia, electrolyte disorders, hypotension, hypoxemia, and fluid imbalances can also lead to postoperative delirium and should be ruled out immediately upon the recognition of the patients altered mental status [1, 2]. This can be achieved through checking electrolyte levels, magnesium, phosphate, calcium, arterial blood gas, hemoglobin level, blood cultures, urine culture, urinalysis, and a chest X-ray [6, 7]. The clinician must remember infection presents differently in the elderly population and may not present with leukocytosis and fever, but may present primarily with delerium [7]. Fluid status as well as overall nutritional status should be checked as well and corrected if need be [6]. The above parameters (electrolytes, oxygenation, etc.,) should be optimized upon recognition of postoperative delirium to begin supportive care and encourage expeditious recovery [6].

Medications and polypharmacy also contribute to postoperative delirium [7]. Anticholinergic medications and benzodiazepines should be avoided when possible [2]. Anticholinergic pharmaceuticals, as well as those drugs with anticholinergic side effects, are well known to contribute to postoperative delirium. However, those patients taking benzodiazepines prior to surgery must be kept on them in the postoperative period to prevent benzodiazepine withdrawal, which can also cause delirium [6]. Other medications known to contribute to delirium include: "cimetidine, corticosteroids, diphenhydramine, belladonna, promethazine, warfarin, narcotics, and antiparkinsonian drugs" as well as morphine [7]. These medications should be minimized when possible. Poor postoperative pain control can also contribute to postoperative delirium and should be prevented [6].

Once postoperative delirium has been diagnosed, patient safety becomes paramount. Those patients with hyperactive or mixed delirium will be prone to pull at lines and tubes [7]. Those patients with hypoactive delirium may wander around or even out of their hospital room, unaware of what he/she is doing [7]. Delirious patients are also at risk of falling and may be unable to protect themselves from themselves [7]. These patients should be monitored more closely with one-to-one surveillance or transfer to a higher acuity setting such as a step down unit or ICU [7]. If initial maneuvers to calm the patient fail and the patient continues to be a danger to themselves, restraints and pharmacologic therapy should be instituted [7]. Haldol, the pharmacologic therapy of choice for delirium, may help keep the patient protected from falling or hurting themselves as a result of delirium [2, 6, 7]. Haldol dosing is dependent upon patient placement in the hospital [7]. Those patients in the ICU should receive a loading dose of 2 mg intravenous with another 2 mg given every 15–20 min until the delirium abates [7]. Once controlled, the delirium should be prophylaxed with scheduled doses. Once on the ward, Haldol should be initially dosed at 1–2 mg with 0.25–0.5 mg every 4 hours [7]. The side effects of this medication are extrapyramidal side effects and prolonged QT syndrome. Periodic EKG's should be monitored while the patient is on this medication [7]. Also, any preoperative metabolic abnormalities, especially those involving sodium, should be corrected prior to surgery if possible [2, 6].

Postoperative Cognitive Dysfunction

Postoperative Cognitive Dysfunction, or postoperative memory or thought impairment, difficult with social integration and \ or executive function slowing of information processing speed, language impairment, and changes in personality, have been described more and more frequently among the elderly population [6, 8, 9]. This symptom complex manifests as difficulty multitasking, short-term memory problems, attention or focusing problems, and trouble "finding words [8]." POCD does not involve alterations in sensorium or consciousness like delirium and also tends to be longer lasting. POCD leads to difficulty in maintaining activities of daily living and tends to affect the patient after he/she is discharged from the hospital, unlike delirium which is mainly an intra-hospital event [8]. POCD results in longer hospital stays, more nursing care, increased cost, and may increase mortality.

The majority of research on POCD has been in the field of cardiac surgery where up to 50–80% of patients may experience POCD, up to 20–60% of these patients may continue to experience POCD months after surgery [6, 8]. The incidence of POCD in those patients undergoing major noncardiac surgery is 23% among 60–69 year-olds and 29% in those patients over age 70. Up to 14% of patients older than 70 continued to have symptoms of POCD 3 months after surgery [8]. Up to 1% of POCD patients may have POCD symptoms last over 1 year from the date of surgery [8].

Severity of surgery also contributes to POCD. Those elderly patients undergoing minor surgery experienced POCD at a rate of 7% [8]. Patients who underwent surgery and were discharged home the same day also had a low incidence of POCD [8].

POCD is a multi-factorial disorder with poorly understood risk factors, but potential causes include age, type of surgery, anesthetic drugs used, decreased preoperative cognitive status, infection, preoperative medications, preoperative depression, co-morbid conditions, intraoperative hypothermia, intraoperative hypotension, intraoperative hypoxia, intraoperative abnormalities in blood glucose, and duration of surgery [6, 8, 9]. However, age is clearly the most important component of POCD [8].

The diagnosis and existence of POCD is clear, however, the exact causation is still being studied. There are several current theories attempting to explain the occurrence of POCD. One such hypothesis is linked to cognitive reserve, where increased reserve may be protective of POCD. This theory is born out of evidence that patients with higher educational level have less POCD [8]. However, it is unclear whether the protection comes directly from higher education or a difference in those patients' brains that pursue higher levels of education. Other theories include the type of anesthetic gas used, however, these theories have been opposed by several studies showing type of gas may not contribute to POCD [8]. However, further studies have shown anesthetic agents can affect postoperative cognitive function, but the deficits rarely last beyond 2 weeks and some agents may even be neuroprotective [8].

Intraoperative hypoxia and hypotension were once thought to contribute to POCD [8]. However, current studies show POCD isn't prevented by guiding oxygen therapy by pulse-oximetry [8, 9]. Studies also show perioperative hypotension, determined by mean arterial pressures, likely does not contribute to POCD [8, 9]. Intraoperative hyperventilation and hypocapnia seem to cause prolonged reaction times and may contribute to POCD [9]. Interestingly, it appears the type of anesthesia may have no affect on POCD, but debate among the literature exists [6, 9]. It is difficult to isolate the type of anesthesia as a cause because controlling for all other surgical factors such as blood pressure can be difficult [9].

As previously mentioned, POCD incidence is dependent on degree of surgery which leads investigators to examine surgery as the cause of POCD [8]. Surgery causes an inflammatory response leading to cytokine release and neuroendocrine hormone release. The surgical stress response is less pronounced in patients undergoing minor surgery [8]. There are reports of inflammatory mediators and cortisol levels being related to delayed functional recovery [8].

The assessment and treatment for POCD mirrors that of assessing cognitive status in the nonoperative patient. These tests include the mini-mental status exam, clock drawing test, and list learning test [8].

As with most other complications, prevention is best the form of treatment. Preventing hypothermia, perioperative hypotension, oxygen therapy, proper pain control, emotional support, and frequent assessments are the best ways to prevent POCD

[8]. Currently, there are no treatment guidelines for POCD and there is no evidence to suggest treating POCD once diagnosed has any effect on the outcome [6].

Urinary Tract Infection

Urinary tract infection (UTI) in the elderly may manifest differently when compared to younger patients as the only symptom may be confusion [2]. Also, many symptoms of UTI may be chronic in this population and discerning symptoms of the aging urinary tract from those of infection may be difficult. Patients may also present with symptoms comparable to their younger counterparts such as urgency, dysuria, and frequency [10]. Those patients with indwelling catheters may not have these symptoms [10]. Not to mention, assessing these symptoms is quite difficult in those patients with cognitive deficiency and may delay diagnosis [10]. Altered sensorium, agitation, further cognitive decline, restlessness, confusion, falls, lethargy, and emotional instability may also indicate pain in this population, which should be further evaluated as suprapubic pain, costovertebral angle pain, and/or flank pain may be secondary to UTI. Changes in urine character may also indicate UTI [10]. Urine may become cloudy and foul smelling, while this is not diagnostic of UTI, it is certainly an indication for further examination [10]. New onset gross hematuria can also be alarming in the postoperative period. There are numerous causes for this including recent instrumentation, indwelling catheter, bladder cancer, and infection as well as several others [10]. However, new onset hematuria in the postoperative patient that presents well after the Foley catheter was placed or removed merits further examination. New onset urinary incontinence can also be a sign of UTI and should prompt further evaluation with urinalysis and culture [10]. The populations at increased risk of presenting with vague or minimal symptoms are those with indwelling catheters, who are incontinent at baseline, receiving analgesics or antipyretics, immunocompromised, and/or cognitively impaired [10].

Less specific symptoms may also be caused by UTI in the elderly population. Fever may be the only indicator of UTI in this population as well and a urinalysis with culture is a standard part of the postoperative fever evaluation. The patient with UTI may also present with hypotension and/or tachycardia [10]. Tachypnea, rales, respiratory distress, nausea, vomiting, and abdominal pain can also be symptoms of UTI in this population [10]. Indwelling foley catheters are an obvious risk factor for UTI [2]. Elderly patients may be more likely to have a catheter secondary to hindered mobility, incontinence, and medication-induced retention [2]. Foley catheters should be removed as soon as possible to minimize the risk of UTI.

Falls

Risk factors for falls include age, cognitive impairment, impaired mobility, and functional impairment [11]. Again, the best way to treat falls in this population is to prevent them. Cognitive impairment as well as prevention thereof has been thoroughly discussed in this chapter. Impaired mobility and functional impairment can be prevented by exercise, early mobilization, and balance training [11].

Frailty

Frailty puts patients at risk for nearly all of the above postoperative complications and a thorough understanding of this concept in the elderly patient is essential. Frailty is a syndrome in elderly patients where decreased reserve, both cognitive and physical, and compensatory mechanisms make the patient more likely to have complications [5, 12]. Frailty puts patients at risk for falls, disability, death, and hospitalization. The symptomatology of frailty remains fairly undefined, but the fact the syndrome exists does not [12]. "Frailty is characterized by a decline in overall health as evidenced by a mass of impairments, such as symptoms, signs, disease, or disability [12]." One system to diagnose frailty uses unintentional weight loss, slow walking speed, self-reported exhaustion, low physical activity, and weakness. In this system, patients with three of these symptoms are considered frail. Up to 20–30% of patients over 75 may have frailty [12]. Another metric to diagnose frailty uses decreased grip strength, self-reported exhaustion, unintentional weight loss of over 4.5 kg in 1 year, slow walking speed, and low physical activity to categorize patients [13]. Once patients reach age 80, most of them will have frailty. This syndrome dramatically increases mortality (18% vs. 4% in the non frail elderly) and likely morbidity [12].

In the postoperative patient, frailty leads to more complications, increased length of stay, and increased likelihood of being discharged to a rehabilitation facility rather than to home, Fig. 6.2 [12, 13]. These patients also are more likely to develop postoperative delirium. Frailty puts patients at increased risk for deep venous thrombosis in the postoperative period secondary to increased D-dimer and factor VIII levels that increase with age as well as in the postoperative state by inflammatory mediators, Fig. 6.2 [12]. This population is also less mobile which sets them up for a DVT, and, therefore, intermittent pneumatic compression devices should be used [12]. For patients who have mild to moderate risk of DVT, low-dose unfractionated heparin 5,000 units twice daily or low molecular weight heparin <3,400 units daily should be used. For those patients at high risk, low dose unfractionated heparin 5,000 units three times per day or low molecular weight heparin >3,400 units daily should be used [12].

Sarcopenia, loss of muscle mass, is of vital concern in this population as its presence leads to decreased mobility as well as strength in an already weakened population. Therefore, this population should be involved in early mobilization programs and postoperative physical therapy programs [12]. A nutrition team should also be involved to help optimize the patients' diet to prevent muscle loss and if patients are unable to tolerate oral feeding, tube feeds or parenteral feeds should be initiated [12].

Frailty can be used as a prognostic factor as well. Those patients who exhibit frailty have higher mortality rates, hospitalization rates, and decreased functional

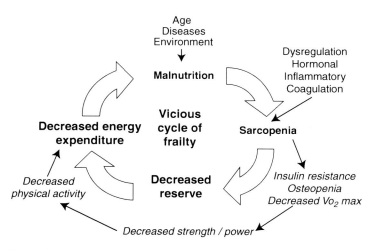

Fig. 6.2 Cycle of frailty. Adapted from McDermid et al. [13]

outcomes [13]. A multifocal approach, including nutrition, physical activity, and psychiatry, is needed to treat and prevent frailty. However, the extent to which we can measure and use frailty to enhance clinical outcomes remains unanswered [13].

References

1. Jin F, Chung F. Minimizing perioperative adverse events in the elderly. Br J Anaesth. 2001;87:608–24.
2. Beliveau MM, Multach M. Perioperative care for the elderly patient. Med Clin North Am. 2003;87:273–89.
3. Story DA. Postoperative complications in elderly patients and their significance for long-term prognosis. Curr Opin Anaesthesiol. 2008;21:375–9.
4. Berman AR. Pulmonary embolism in the elderly. Clin Geriatr Med. 2001;17:107–30.
5. Colloca G, Santoro M, Gambassi G. Age-related physiologic changes and perioperative management of elderly patients. Surg Oncol. 2010;19:124–30.
6. Bekker AY, Weeks EJ. Cognitive function after anaesthesia in the elderly. Best Pract Res Clin Anaesthesiol. 2003;17:259–72.
7. Robinson TN, Eiseman B. Postoperative delirium in the elderly: diagnosis and management. Clin Interv Aging. 2008;3:351–5.
8. Ramaiah R, Lam AM. Postoperative cognitive dysfunction in the elderly. Anesthesiol Clin. 2009;27:485–96.
9. Dodds C, Allison J. Postoperative cognitive deficit in the elderly surgical patient. Br J Anaesth. 1998;81:449–62.
10. Midthun SJ. Criteria for urinary tract infection in the elderly: variables that challenge nursing assessment. Urol Nurs. 2004;24:157–62, 166–9, 186; quiz 170.

11. Cicerchia M, Ceci M, Locatelli C, Gianni W, Repetto L. Geriatric syndromes in peri-operative elderly cancer patients. Surg Oncol. 2010;19:131–9.
12. Brown NA, Zenilman ME. The impact of frailty in the elderly on the outcome of surgery in the aged. Adv Surg. 2010;44:229–49.
13. McDermid RC, Stelfox HT, Bagshaw SM. Frailty in the critically ill: a novel concept. Crit Care. 2011;15:301.

Chapter 7
Use of Adjunctive Services

Mary Ann Forciea

Introduction

Older patients present for care with a wide range of functional abilities, reside in a spectrum of locations, and require a variety of supportive services for care after active treatment. This chapter is designed to help you

- Understand the functional requirements for transfer or discharge to different sites of senior living
- Understand the support services available to older patients wherever their discharge location
- Improve your ability to gather historical or medical information about older patients
- Improve your communication with outside caregivers to improve after-care

Sites of Care (See Table 7.1)

The commonly encountered residential locations of older patients will be reviewed in this section, with attention to functional status requirements for that site, medical/nursing support available, medicare coverage considerations, and monthly costs.

M.A. Forciea (✉)
Division of Geriatric Medicine, Department of Medicine,
University of Pennsylvania Health System, Philadelphia, PA 19104, USA
e-mail: forciea@mail.med.upenn.edu

T.J. Guzzo et al. (eds.), *Primer of Geriatric Urology*, DOI 10.1007/978-1-4614-4773-3_7,   77
© Springer Science+Business Media New York 2013

Table 7.1 Characteristics of sites of care

	Home	Assisted living/personal care home	Rehabilitation facility	Nursing home-short stay	Nursing home—long-term stay
Functional status	Independent[a]	Independent in ADLs, assistance with IADLs[a]	May be dependent in some ADLs, IADLs	Dependent in ADLs, IADLs	Dependent in ADLs, IADLs
Nursing staff	None (visiting nurse services available)	Most have limited daytime nursing staff coverage	Nurses, all shifts	Nurses, all shifts	Nurses, all shifts
Physician visits	Office visits Home care visits	Office visits Home care visits	Facility MDs available daily	Facility MDs/NPs see patient within 72 h of admission, then every 30 days. Urgent visits variably available. 24-h telephone coverage.	Facility MDs/NPs see patient within 72 h of admission, then every 30 days, then every 90 days, then every 60 days. Urgent visits variably available. 24-h telephone coverage
Medicare coverage	Office visits, home care visits, short-term skilled VN agency services	Office visits, home care, short-term, skilled VN agency services	Covered	First 21 days covered, then decreasing coverage	Not covered May transition to Medicaid coverage
Average monthly cost 2011		$4,000–6,000			$10,000–12,000 for private payment

ADLs Activities of Daily Living (bathing, toilet use, dressing, eating, mobility); IADLs (shopping, travel, financial management, telephone, cooking, taking medications, laundry, housekeeping); VN visiting nurse; MD physician; NP nurse practitioner

[a]In many cases, can purchase additional services to remain at this level in spite of increasing deficits

Table 7.2 Functional status

Activities of daily living (ADLs)	Instrumental activities of daily living (IADLs)	
Bathing	Cooking	Laundry
Dressing	Shopping	Housekeeping
Toilet use	Travel	Telephone use
Eating	Managing finances	
Mobility	Managing medications	
Transfers from bed to chair		

Home Care

The vast majority of older patients reside in their own homes. These patients, either on their own or with the support of family, manage their own needs, and are independent in Activities of Daily Living (ADLs) and Instrumental Activities of Daily Living (IADLs)—see Table 7.2.

Patients should have primary care practitioners and make office visits; many areas of the country have house call practitioners who can visit homebound seniors to provide ongoing primary care [1]. The American Academy of Home Care Physicians has a website with access listings for house call providers (http:\\www.aahcp.org).

Older patients with temporary needs for nursing oversight following a hospitalization or outpatient procedure can be referred to a *visiting nurse agency*. These multi-service organizations provide short-term skilled nursing services (wound care, medication monitoring and adjustment, home assessment, and teaching), rehabilitation services from physical, occupational, and speech therapy, social work, and some specialty nursing services such as wound care and ostomy care. Some agencies have expanded to provide home intravenous support and nutrition support; these agencies are often hospital owned and managed. For residents who require ADL support, temporary home health aides can be provided for short periods. The costs of care are usually covered by Medicare, but may require pre-authorization in Medicare managed care. The duration of care extends as long as the skilled care needs can be documented: as long as progress towards goals of care is being made. Once the patient has stabilized or reached a plateau in status, services are withdrawn. Visiting Nurse Agency episodes of care rarely exceed 6 weeks.

For patients who require long-term supportive care services at home, some special programs have been developed. Patients and families may privately pay companions or home health aides to provide care. In many areas of the country, assistance is available to help support patients and families in need of services at home. These programs are supported mainly through Medicaid programs of the states and vary widely. The programs are coordinated by a network of *Area Agencies on Aging* which are located in every county and provide information and access to state and federal programs available in a region. Local agencies can be accessed through the website of the National Association of Area Agencies on Aging: http:\\www.n4a.org

An interesting innovation in the care of the frail elderly has been the development of *Programs of All-Inclusive Care of the Elderly* (*PACE*) programs throughout the nation [2]. These programs offer to Medicare/Medicaid eligible seniors a coordinated menu of medical and social programs at specialized sites. Because PACE sites are equivalent to managed care and are capitated for each member, sites often develop specialized referral networks for their patients.

Seniors who find the maintenance of their homes too difficult can opt for *senior housing* in specialized buildings which also offer increased security. Rent may be income-linked; many of these buildings are built with federal support for low-income elderly. Larger facilities may offer some social work access, but no health or social services are mandated in these buildings, and the residents are expected to be independent in their apartments.

Assisted Living Facilities/Personal Care Homes

The fastest growing segment of housing for older people is the *Assisted Living Facility* (*ALF*). These often "for-profit" buildings offer apartments of various sizes as well as dining rooms providing daily meals, and often some program of activities. Residents are expected to be independent within their apartment (ADL independent). Many offer housekeeping, laundry, and medication oversight as additional charges. Some facilities offer "memory" programs with additional activities and oversight—these specialized areas are usually more expensive. Residents or families are responsible for obtaining medical care which is usually provided in an outside physician's office. State regulation of these facilities ranges from nonexistent to nascent; services may vary widely from state to state, and even county to county. Costs are generally covered by patients and families themselves; some states are beginning to allow Medicaid payments to ALFs. While these facilities are generally attractive physically (resembling apartments rather than nursing homes), these sites generally cannot meet the life-long requirements for care for residents with progressive illnesses such as dementia. Residents will need either to relocate again to a nursing home when they become ADL dependent, or purchase increasingly expensive amounts of care in the ALF.

Personal care homes also provide housing (usually in a shared bedroom) and meals for lower income patients. In most states, Medicaid will cover most of the costs of care for this level of service. Again, medical care is provided off site in a physician's office; no nursing care is provided as a routine. Some homes will assist in medication oversight but many do not.

Rehabilitation Facilities

Older patients recovering from an acute illness or hospitalization can be referred to short stay *rehabilitation* facilities if they need physical, occupational, or speech therapy, and can tolerate at least 3 h of therapy daily. These facilities aim at preparing patients for discharge to their homes. Stays are covered by Medicare. Older acute-care patients may be declined by these facilities on referral because of patients' cardiopulmonary limitations on endurance, or on cognitive abilities to carry over each day's therapy to the next day. Cognitively intact older patients who were functionally independent on admission should not be routinely excluded from consideration for referral to rehabilitation facilities.

Long-term acute convalescent units (LTACs) have developed to serve inpatients with highly skilled but relatively stable needs such as long-term antibiotic therapy or ventilator-dependent patients recovering from acute illnesses. Stays are usually Medicare approved, but may require pre-authorization.

Nursing Facilities

Elderly patients who need short-term stays in *Nursing Facilities* for skilled care following illness or treatment may receive that care under Medicare. Nursing and rehabilitation services are provided as long as the patient is making progress toward defined skilled care goals. Medicare pays in full for up to 21 days of skilled care; medicare pays a decreasing proportion of costs of care for longer stays if skilled care goal progress continues to be met. At the point that patients have returned to baseline or have stopped making progress, they must be discharged home or become long stay patients at a long-term nursing facility. In many facilities, this may involve a transfer from one area of the facility to another.

Long-term care in a nursing facility provides support for both ADL and IADLs. Nurses are available on all shifts, although at a reduced ratio from that seen in hospital settings. Physicians visit the facility based on the number of patients for whom they provide care. A medical director oversees care and sets protocols for care. Admitting orders are often telephoned to covering physicians; a newly admitted patient must be seen by his physician within 72 h of admission. Both because of the increasing acuity of patients admitted to long-term care, and to the sporadic nature of physician visits, some larger facilities are adding Nurse Practitioners to their staff [3]. Long-term care in nursing facilities is privately paid by patients/families, or by Medicaid programs. Quality comparisons for all medicare certified facilities are available at http:\\www.medicare.gov under "nursing home compare" A very small percentage of long-term care is covered by long-term care insurance.

Hospice

Hospice services are available to Medicare patients who wish to shift the focus of their care to quality of life, and who are felt to have less than 6 months of life remaining. The original focus of many hospice programs was on the end of life care of cancer patients; more modern programs have expanded to include all the major late life diagnoses such as dementia, heart failure, renal failure, and COPD. Because of their expertise in palliation of symptoms, many hospice programs have opened palliative care options which do not exclude active treatment during care. The focus on expected duration of care has also changed somewhat; patients are evaluated on admission and at regular intervals; patients who stabilize or improve on the hospice approach to care are transferred back to regular care with remaining hospice benefits placed on hold. The majority of hospice care in the United States is provided in patients' homes. Inpatient hospice units are becoming more available in the United States, and can offer respite to families or help with more difficult palliative needs. Hospice care provided to residents of nursing facilities is a new venue for hospice services with additional palliative care options for these residents and their families.

Continuing Care Retirement Communities

The past two decades have seen growth in the development of "communities" which provide housing for older people who are independent in their functional needs, but also include assisted living, and nursing facility level care for residents as they age in place. Both non-for-profit and profit models of such care exist. The models can be tightly controlled with a single administration managing medical care and transitions of care between levels, or may provide property management with individual accountability for health care. Since many of these communities require substantial entry fees, care in investigation of community management, finances, and social activities are necessary prior to entry.

General Considerations

Office-Based care

Older patients seen in the office setting will most likely be living at home either independently or supported by family. Special considerations for these older patients are listed in Table 7.3. Telephone "menus" should always feature a "speak to office staff" option mentioned early in the menu. Older office patients may have difficulty with access to the office, if long walks from parking or drop off areas are required. Due to the high incidence of multiple chronic conditions, more time may be required to satisfactorily complete the office visit. Patients and families who require temporary skilled nursing services such as wound care, ostomy care, or medication monitoring should be referred to local Visiting Nurse Agencies.

Patients who are residing in Nursing Facilities can be a special challenge in the office: they may arrive on stretchers or wheelchairs (requiring more space in the waiting area), have complex medical issues, and require facility forms for completion. These frail patients may be unable to tolerate long waiting times, or have pick-up schedules arranged prior to the visit. Office staff should ask about plans for

Table 7.3 Office-based care of older patients

- Allow time for information from a secondary source (in addition to the patient)
    - Spouse
    - Family
    - Outside records (nursing facility, assisted living facility)
- Ask patients/family to repeat back important information
    - Test results
    - Treatment plans
- Write down important information for patient/family to review after the visit
- Refer patients to local visiting nurse agencies for temporary skilled care needs such as wound care, ostomy care teaching, or medication monitoring

Table 7.4 Tips for hospital care of older patients

- In reviewing medications, ask patients which pills they actually take rather than relying solely on electronic lists
- Alternate sources of admitting information for confused older patients:
    - Family members
    - Nursing facility transfer sheets
    - Nursing facility charge nurses
    - Primary care offices
- Work with hospital discharge planning staff from time of admission on options for after-care
- Prepare discharge summary information prior to discharge to accompany patient to nursing facility or for transmission to the primary care office for follow-up care

transportation. Information on diagnoses made, tests ordered, and treatment plans should always be sent back to the facility with the patient after the visit.

Hospital Care (See Table 7.4)

The hospital care of older patients can present many challenges which are discussed in many chapters of this book. This section will focus on information sharing between sites of care for hospitalized older patients.

While the advent and spread of electronic medical records (emr) has been of great benefit to older patients in ease and legibility of medical information, some cautions must be reviewed:

- Some patients may receive care from more than one health system; the emr may be incomplete.
- Medication lists may not correspond to actual medications, doses, or dosing intervals used by the patients. Medication reviews should always be checked with the patient/family on admission.
- Advance Directive status may change over time. Advance Directive status information should be confirmed during the admitting process.

Table 7.5 Tips for safe and effective discharge of patients to nursing facilities

* Write medication or laboratory orders sufficient for 72 h
* Send Rx for new medications, especially narcotics
* Send discharge summary information to both the patient's primary care provider's office and to the admitting physician at the nursing facility

Information gathering on older, newly admitted inpatients can be challenging. If the patients themselves cannot provide complete or reliable information, families or nursing facility staff can be telephoned. If information is needed from the patient's nursing facility, the charge nurse on the floor caring for the patient is often the best source of information.

Successful, efficient patient flow during the process of care requires team management from physicians, nurses, social workers, and discharge planners. The entire team should be aware of possible discharge needs for the patient from the time of admission, with updates as clinical situations change. Patients and families should be included in this planning process as early as possible.

The information regarding the hospital stay contained in the Discharge Summary should be shared with responsible providers as soon as possible on discharge. Ideally, summaries should accompany patients who are being discharged to other health facilities such as nursing homes or rehabilitation facilities. Summaries should be transmitted to Primary Care offices so that providers are prepared to participate in needed follow-up care. Critical, short-term treatment or assessment needs should be telephoned to these providers.

Optimal discharge arrangements for patients being transferred to long-term care (nursing or rehabilitation facilities) have some special requirements (See Table 7.5). Patients are being transferred from one team of providers (hospital) to another team (long-term care facility). All members of the team need to transfer information on diagnoses, test/procedure results, pending results, and plans for ongoing care. This information is shared in a variety of forms: state-mandated transfer forms (usually completed by nurses), discharge orders and summaries (usually completed by physicians, nurse practitioners, or physicians' assistants), social work, and rehabilitation assessments. Urgent or critical information should be shared by telephone contact at the time of transfer.

In most states, upon arrival in a nursing home following a hospital discharge, the patient will receive a thorough nursing assessment. Admitting orders, written by the discharging hospital physician, will be telephoned to the new nursing home physician for approval, that new physician will see the patient within 72 h of admission to the facility. Following that initial visit, nursing facility-based practitioners will see the patient monthly for the first 3 months, then every 2 months thereafter. Urgent visits for changes in medical condition are made at any time as needed.

Conclusions

Effective care of older patients requires an understanding of the network of support services and locations of care which may be required during recovery. Assessment of function is critical to appropriate planning for treatment and recovery. Options for increased care for patients in their homes in the community are usually coordinated through local Visiting Nurse Agencies. Short-term rehabilitation stays can be accomplished in rehabilitation facilities or in nursing facilities. Long-term care can be provided at home or in nursing facilities. For older, frail patients in home the burdens of treatment have begun to outweigh possible benefits, options for palliative hospice care at home or in an inpatient hospice should be offered to patients and their families.

References

1. Landers SH. Why health care is going home. N Engl J Med. 2010;363:1690–91.
2. Program of All-Inclusive Care for the Elderly. Center for Medicare and Medicaid Services. 2011. Available from http://www.cms.hhs.gov/PACE. Accessed April 2011.
3. Levy C, Palat SI, Kramer AM. Physician practice patterns in nursing homes. J Am Med Dir Assoc. 2007;8(9):558–67.

Chapter 8
Urology in the Nursing Home

George W. Drach and Edna P. Schwab

We, a urologist and a geriatrician, conduct patient Grand Rounds (some personal and some chart-based) at our Philadelphia Veterans Administration Nursing Home on a monthly basis. Why? Because we find that this patient group, men and women confined to a long-term care (LTC) environment, harbor many urologic problems that require consultation and treatment. Several authors have recommended special attention to urology in the nursing home [1–3]. In particular, we agree with Pranikoff [1] that the major problems encountered in the nursing home are voiding dysfunction and incontinence and its consequences, indwelling catheters and their management, asymptomatic bacteriuria, symptomatic urinary tract infection (UTI), hematuria, and considerations of sexuality [4]. We add to that our frequent encounters with the problems of management of prostate cancer and stone disease in the chronically ill or bed-bound and often demented patient. Of course, with the decline in numbers of nursing home patients over the past years (Fig. 8.1), some of the urologic problems of the LTC patient will be transferred to the home-bound patient, but the problems continue to exist.

This chapter deals with each of these issues presented above. First we will discuss the problem of true prevalence of incontinence in the nursing home patient. According to Anger et al. [5], incontinence of newly admitted nursing home residents is greatly under-reported and is said to be in the range of 1–2%. Their investigation of a National Nursing Home Survey revealed that over 50% of females

G.W. Drach (✉)
Department of Surgery, Perelman Center for Advanced Medicine,
Hospital of the University of Pennsylvania, Philadelphia, PA 19104, USA
e-mail: drachg@uphs.upenn.edu

E.P. Schwab
Department of Medicine, Division of Geriatrics, Hospital of the University of Pennsylvania,
Philadelphia Veterans Administration Medical Center, Philadelphia, PA 19104, USA

T.J. Guzzo et al. (eds.), *Primer of Geriatric Urology*, DOI 10.1007/978-1-4614-4773-3_8,   87
© Springer Science+Business Media New York 2013

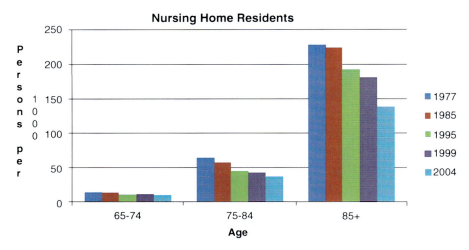

Fig. 8.1 Gradual decrease in the number of nursing home residents of all ages from 1977 to 2004. Adapted from Centers for Disease Control and Prevention. 2012. National Center for Health Statistics. Health Data Interactive. Available from: http:\\www.cdc.gov/nchs/hdi.htm. Accessed 2 Apr 2012

had "difficulty controlling urination" or needed assistance in using the toilet. Klausner and Vapnek [6] carried this observation further by evaluating female and male nursing home residents and pointed out that the incidence in females exceeds that in males by a ratio of 2:1. Shih et al. [7] analyzed the labor costs associated with incontinence in nursing homes and estimated that individual added costs per patient per day were $13.57 or nearly $5,000 annually. Incontinence therefore represents one of the greatest urologic problems in the nursing home. How is it dealt with?

Voiding Dysfunction and Catheters

Multiple problems may lead to incontinence in these patients: urethral sphincter weakness, UTI, urinary urgency or involuntary bladder contractions, bladder atony and/or overflow incontinence associated with obstruction. Hopefully the primary causes associated with the abnormal voiding function have been defined, but often "shotgun" methods (anti-muscarinic drugs or catheterization) begin without full evaluation. Foremost amongst these is use of bladder catheterization for the control of incontinence [8]. Newman et al. point out that reduction in catheter use to treat incontinence is one of the mandates of the Centers for Medicare and Medicaid Services (CMS) issued in 2005. This, of course, helps in decreasing the related incidences of UTI, urethral erosion, urethritis and epididymitis and especially in females, catheter expulsion. If the indwelling urethral catheter does become the method chosen, the next questions are: [1] how often should it be changed, especially if one is to reduce the risk of symptomatic urinary infection and [2] how should the catheter be cared for? These dilemmas present some of the strongest reasons for urologists to be well acquainted with nursing home care.

Priefer et al. [9] performed an interesting study of patients in a VA Nursing home. Catheters were changed in two random groups: group 1 only for acute infection or catheter obstruction (7 men), and group 2 on a regular monthly schedule as well as for infection or obstruction (10 men). Six of the former group (86%) developed symptomatic UTI while only three of ten in group two did so (30%). Obviously, this was a limited study, but it seems to corroborate the usual advice to change indwelling urethral catheters on a monthly basis.

Nursing homes usually have available noninvasive devices for measurement of bladder residual urine volume. These assist the urologist in decisions about degree of obstruction or inadequate bladder emptying. If increased residual exists, then conservative treatment methods may lead to a satisfactory resolution, but again, an indwelling catheter is frequently attempted as the first intervention, rather than preferred alternate techniques such as sterile or clean-intermittent-catheterization (CIC) [10]. If the patient can perform CIC, then that is better for them. If it must be done by nursing personnel, the time requirements may seem excessive, but the proven decrease in symptomatic UTI for intermittent over indwelling catheterization pleads for the use of CIC [11]. Of course, if increased residual is related to outlet obstruction, some procedural intervention to relieve obstruction may be necessary. In the absence of obstruction, other simple procedures such as timed voiding, double voiding or expedited access to a commode may be the only interventions needed [3, 12].

When problems such as recurrent urethral erosion appear in a patient, the question of inserting a suprapubic tube arises. Our judgment often results from the success or failure of previous attempts to correct the voiding dysfunction: relief of outlet obstruction by surgical intervention in the up and about patient, intermittent catheterization in any patient where the obstruction or bladder atony cannot be overcome, use of condom catheters where incontinence exists without obstruction. When all these interventions that may be tried have failed, then perhaps a test of suprapubic catheterization may be performed with a percutaneous insertion under ultrasound guidance [13]. If this provides adequate improvement, a more permanent retention catheter can be placed by gradual size increases.

One of the complications that the suprapubic catheter helps to avoid is the meatal or urethral erosion sometimes associated with indwelling catheterization (Fig. 8.2). But another way to avoid the complication is to conduct educational programs for the staff charged with catheter management [14]. Proper draping of the drainage tube to avoid urethral tension, and attention to re-draping when the patient is repositioned resulted in a decreased number of these events in our experience.

Fig. 8.2 Severe urethral erosion associated with indwelling urinary catheter (from Juthani-Mehta [15]; with permission)

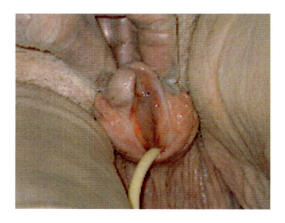

Asymptomatic Bacteriuria and UTI

Another of the significant problems encountered in the nursing home patient is the presence of bacteria in the urine: asymptomatic or symptomatic? We know that this is common in conjunction with long-term indwelling catheter, but it also occurs in the catheter free patient. What is the significance of these bacteria? Juthani-Mehta [15] published an extensive review on this subject and presented precise requirements for diagnosis of asymptomatic bacteriuria versus UTI. One question that always arises is the validity of using a dipstick to detect infection. Perhaps the most important component here is that a negative dipstick strongly mitigates against bacteriuria and thus against UTI. However, any dipstick positivity must be followed by a properly collected urine specimen for culture.

Notably, the incidence of asymptomatic bacteriuria increases with increasing age and thus (from our Fig. 8.1) in community or nursing home populations, being barely 1–2% until age 65, but over 6% thereafter in community dwelling elderly. For those patients in LTC institutions, the prevalence is greater than 15%. Sometimes this finding of bacteriuria is associated with symptoms of true infection: fever, painful urination, and so forth. But these symptoms may not clearly diagnose true UTI: "To date no constellation of symptoms is identified in older adults who have bacteriuria that can distinguish symptomatic from asymptomatic patients reliably in all situations" [15]. However, in the presence of symptomatic bacteriuria, presence of at least three of four criteria may be useful in deciding to treat (Table 8.1).

Hematuria

Another vexing problem seen in the LTC patient is hematuria. This may be found microscopically on routine urinalysis (and remember that to be considered significant by American Urological Assn criteria must be greater that 2

Table 8.1 Help in diagnosing UTI in nursing home patients (presence of at least 3 of 4 criteria) [15]

Fever greater than 100.4 °F
New or increased burning on urination, frequency, or urgency
New flank or suprapubic pain or tenderness
Change in character of urine and/or worsening of mental or functional status

RBC/HPF in at least two microscopic examinations of adequately collected urinary specimens) [16] or perhaps grossly present and noted by the patient or nursing personnel. Dipstick positivity for hematuria is not adequate for defining true hematuria. In any case, this drives the urologist toward standard evaluation including collection of specimen for cytology, anatomic imaging, and cystoscopic examination. However, questions always arise about the necessity of such procedures in the bed-ridden demented patient or one with multiple co-morbidities for whom no significant intervention would be considered. In such situations, one must consult with responsible family or guardian or other individual with health care power of attorney.

Sexuality

One of the most poignant presentations of this subject occurs in the fictional book by F. Scott Peck, MD entitled "A Bed by the Window" [4]. This is the story of a LTC patient assigned to the inside bed of a double bedded room. Her greatest desire is to ultimately move to the window bed so that she can see the outside view every day. But throughout this book one is shown the various day-to-day activities within the LTC facility—and that includes sexual innuendo and encounters amongst patients and staff. Pranikoff has stated that "Sexuality in nursing home residents is neglected and often suppressed by staff," yet he continues by saying "surveys confirm that sexual interest and the need to show affection to another person remains important for nursing home residents." Certainly problems can occur when one patient pursues another, who may be partly or fully demented, or if a member of the staff pursues a patient. He [1] encourages nursing homes to educate staff and to establish reasonable rules to allow appropriate relationships.

Urinary Stone Disease

Use of long-term indwelling urethral catheters leads to urinary infections as noted above [17]. Even the presence of a suprapubic catheter increases the risk of formation of bladder stone [13]. These infections result in increased incidence of cystitis and pyelonephritis [18], with the result that infection-related stones occur. In addition, those patients with a genetic predisposition toward metabolic urinary stone disease continue to develop stones if in the LTC facility. Management of LTC patients with stone disease is complicated by lack of nearby imaging facilities or poor control of pain. If the stone is "quiet," it may be detected only because of the investigation stimulated by discovery of hematuria (see above). Fortunately, the advent of minimally invasive techniques for stone removal decrease significantly the risk to the chronically ill patient, but even at a minimum, any such procedure requires transfer to a fully equipped hospital.

Prostatic and Other Genito-Urinary Cancers

Since the incidence of prostate cancer continues to increase with age and with the increased number of elderly men, it is inevitable that more LTC male patients will have prostate cancer. Techniques such as radical prostatectomy may or may not be indicated for the LTC patient, but more conservative methods such as radioactive seed insertion or external beam radiation may provide adequate therapy if the patient or responsible surrogate express desire for treatment. Of course, the concept of "watchful waiting" may always be instituted, especially for those with limited life spans or with many co-morbidities [19]. Sometimes the patient or surrogate may urge surgical intervention of some type against the urologist's advice. This event occurred in our experience when a demented, bed-ridden man of 84 years somehow had a PSA performed, and the result was greatly elevated. On examination the prostate was irregular and hard. Most of us would consider this presumptive evidence of prostate cancer. When these findings were discussed with his wife, she insisted that we perform a biopsy to "prove that he had cancer." We explained the multiple and potentially serious complications that might occur—but the insistence remained. We also pointed out the medical concept that it was not usual to obtain a biopsy if the result—a cancer—was not likely to be treated, as we believed to be the case for this patient. She indicated that if a cancer was found, she wished it to be treated. Prostate cancer of high grade was found, and in agreement with the patient's wife, he was placed on anti-androgen therapy. This clinical story illustrates the difficulty one might have in dealing not only with the patient, but with the patient's surrogate. Yet in counseling this patient's surrogate, it was clear that diagnosis and treatment were strongly desired, in spite of our advice to the contrary [20].

Other urologic cancers such as bladder and kidney increase greatly with increasing age (Chapter 9), so that one must remain alert to these possibilities. Once again, the signal often is hematuria, followed by the complete evaluation. Minimally invasive methods such as partial nephrectomy, or robotic cystectomy and diversion that would not have been possible in the frail elderly LTC patient may now be successfully completed when the operative plan includes all the precautions necessary for the elderly and partly or wholly disabled patient (see Chapters 2 and 5)

Ethics and the Functionally and Cognitively Impaired Patient

The decision to pursue any medical evaluation and treatment for an impaired long-term care resident is very individualized and should be determined by several factors. These include the potential risks vs. benefits of specific diagnostic evaluation and treatment, the surrogate decision maker's wishes or directives of a patient's living will. The purposes are to maintain the patient's present functional and cognitive status as well as their quality of life. For instance, one would likely not pursue an intensive and invasive evaluation of hematuria in a long-term care resident who is moderately to severely demented, lacks functional capacity, and requires complete nursing assistance for all activities of daily living. After discussion of the problem by the medical team and surrogate, a reasonable approach to hematuria in such a patient would be to obtain a urinalysis checking for evidence of infection and cytology for abnormal cells. If infection or abnormal cells were not present, pursuing an evaluation of the prostate, bladder and upper tracts would likely not yield information that would improve the survival and quality of life of this resident. Palliative approaches to any symptoms the resident may express would be provided including pain control with analgesics, bladder irrigation if blood clots obstruct urinary flow or relief of obstruction with an indwelling Foley catheter [21].

Some long-term care residents will have an advance health care directive such as a living will which provides a written statement of their desires regarding life sustaining treatment and other medical care when he/she becomes incompetent. When these document(s) are not available then the health care team will need to discuss risks, benefits, and treatment options with the health care agent or health care power of attorney. If neither is available, then the health care team must provide the best quality of life care available. When possible, good communication between health care providers and any health care agents will lead to a thoughtful and palliative approach to the care of the long-term care resident with end stage disease [22].

Conclusion

Patients in nursing homes, or LTCs, harbor a myriad of urologic problems. Urologists often do not become involved with nursing homes because of distance, difficulty dealing with aged elderly patients, or in dealing with the complex Federal- and Medicare-related regulations. But, as shown throughout this Chapter, patients in nursing homes may have many urologic problems, most of which can be improved by simple and conservative urologic interventions. Communication between the urologist and the nursing home nurses and physicians, and occasional onsite consultations [3], leads to improved urologic care of the patients and therefore their enhanced comfort and quality of life.

References

1. Pranikoff K. Urologic care in long-term facilities. Urol Clin North Am. 1996;23:137–46.
2. Foster LB. Why a urology consultant in a geriatric skilled and LTC facility. Nurs Homes. 1973;22:26–7.
3. Watson RA, Suchak N, Steel K. A doctor in the house: rationale for providing on-site urological consultation to geriatric patients in nursing health care facilities. Urology. 2010;76:277–81.
4. Peck MS. A bed by the window. New York: Bantam Books; 1990.
5. Anger JT, Saigal CS, Pace J, et al. True prevalence of urinary incontinence among female nursing home residents. Urology. 2006;67:281–7.
6. Klausner AP, Vapnek JM. Urinary incontinence in the geriatric population. Mt Sinai J Med. 2003;70:54–61.
7. Shih YC, Hartzema AG, Tolleson-Rinehart S. Labor costs associated with incontinence in long-term care facilities. Urology. 2003;62:442–6.
8. Newman DK, Gaines T, Snare E. Innovation in bladder assessment: use of technology in extended care. J Gerontol Nurs. 2005;31:33–41.
9. Priefer BA, Duthie EH, Gambert SR. Frequency of urinary catheter change and clinical urinary tract infection. Urology. 1982;20:141–2.
10. Newman DK, Willson MM. Review of intermittent catheterization and current best practices. Urol Nurs. 2011;31:12–28.
11. Bennett CJ, Diokno AC. Clean intermittent self-catheterization in the elderly. Urology. 1984;24:43–5.
12. Zimakoff J, Pontoppidan B, Larsen SO, et al. Management of urinary bladder function in Danish hospitals, nursing homes and home care. J Hosp Infect. 1993;24:183–99.
13. Mutsui T, Minami K, Foruno T, et al. Is suprapubic cystostomy on optimal management in high quadriplegics? Eur Urol. 2000;38:434–8.
14. LeBlanc K, Christensen D. Addressing the challenge of providing nursing care for elderly men suffering from urethral erosion. J WOCN. 2005;32:131–4.
15. Juthani-Mehta M. Asymptomatic bacteriuria and urinary tract infection in older adults. Clin Geriatr Med. 2007;23:583–94.
16. Grossfeld GD, Wolf Jr JS, Litwan MS, et al. Asymptomatic microscopic hematuria in adults: summary of AUA best practice policy recommendations. Am Fam Physician. 2001;63:1145–54.
17. Warren JW. Catheter-associated urinary tract infection. Infect Dis Clin North Am. 1997;11:609–22.
18. Warren JW, Muncie HL, Hebel JR, et al. Long-term urethral catheterization increases risk of chronic pyelonephritis and renal inflammation. J Am Geriatr Soc. 1994;42:1286–90.
19. Guzzo TJ, Drach GW. Major urologic problems in geriatrics: assessment and management. Med Clin North Am. 2011;95:253–64.
20. Reuben DB, Cassel CK. Physician stewardship of health care in an era of finite resources. JAMA. 2009;302:2686–94.
21. Klimes R. Nursing Home Admin Ethics. 2012. Available from: http://www.learnwell.org/nursinghomeethics.htm. Accessed 16 Apr 2012.
22. Pennsylvania Health Care Act of 2006. Available from: http://www.pamedsoc.org/MainMenuCategories/Government/LawsAffectingPhysicians/AdvanceDirectives/Act169facts.html. Accessed 16 Apr 2012.

Chapter 9
Urologic Oncology

Matthew J. Resnick and Thomas J. Guzzo

Surgical Considerations in Elderly Cancer Patients

Currently, approximately half of all surgical procedures in the U.S. are performed in patients ≥65 years of age [1]. Furthermore, 50% of new cancer diagnoses are made in patients ≥70 years of age [2]. Many elderly patients have complex physiologic and functional issues which merit consideration when contemplating surgical intervention. The aging process is associated with changes in many organ systems that can impact an elderly patient's ability to withstand and tolerate a major surgical procedure. The cardiac, pulmonary, hepatobiliary, immune, and renal systems all undergo deterioration and loss of physiologic reserve with aging. Knowledge of such changes with regard to perioperative management is essential in the evaluation of the elderly surgical candidate. Renal function decreases with age and serum creatinine is a poor surrogate for glomerular filtration rate (GFR) in elderly patients [3]. Renal drug dose adjustment and proper perioperative fluid balance are essential in attempting to minimize morbidity. Cardiac changes that accompany aging include a lower sensitivity to beta adrenergic modulation, altered calcium regulation, and an overall reduction in ejection fraction [2]. Occult coronary artery disease is not uncommon and a high index of suspicion for underlying cardiac pathology and prompt preoperative cardiology consultation is essential. A decline in immune function in the elderly has two important implications for the urologic surgeon. First, immune decline may predispose individuals to the development and progression of cancer [3]. Altered immunologic function may also lead to an increased susceptibility

M.J. Resnick
Department of Urologic Surgery, Vanderbilt University Medical Center,
Nashville, TN 37232, USA

T.J. Guzzo (✉)
Department of Surgery, Division of Urology, Perelman Center for Advanced Medicine,
Hospital of the University of Pennsylvania, Philadelphia, PA 19104, USA
e-mail: thomas.guzzo@uphs.upenn.edu

T.J. Guzzo et al. (eds.), *Primer of Geriatric Urology*, DOI 10.1007/978-1-4614-4773-3_9,
© Springer Science+Business Media New York 2013

to infection during cancer therapy [3]. A significant reduction in liver volume with aging is also accompanied by an overall decrease in hepatic function, which can have obvious implications when dosing chemotherapeutic agents. Finally, decreased respiratory function from intrinsic lung disease, weakened respiratory musculature, pulmonary vascular disease, or a combination of the three can predispose elderly patients to significant postoperative pulmonary complications [2].

The burden of medical comorbidity frequently impacts clinical decision-making with regard to the pursuit of aggressive oncologic therapy. Comorbidity is also a valuable predictor of perioperative outcome(s). Comorbidity scores are useful in the quantification of surgical risk in the elderly. Several useful scores to assess overall comorbidity include the Cumulative Illness Rating Scale for Geriatrics (CIRS-G), the Charlson Comorbidity Index (CCI) and the American Society of Anesthesiologists Classification (ASA). The CIRS-G and CCI have been validated in elderly populations with less favorable scores found to be associated with increased perioperative morbidity and mortality [4, 5]. In fact, overall comorbidity is a more useful predictor of perioperative outcome than chronologic age alone. Sanchez-Sales et al. recently evaluated outcomes following laparoscopic radical prostatectomy in men ≥ 70 [6]. In this cohort of 297 men, a CCI ≥ 2 was associated with a higher risk of short-term postoperative complications compared those with lower CCI. Similarly, with regard to laparoscopic renal surgery, Guzzo et al. found a CCI ≥ 2 to be a significant predictor of perioperative complications in patients ≥ 75 years age [7].

While comorbidity is an important indicator of outcome, it generally does not take into account overall global functioning. Careful preoperative attention to functional status in the elderly surgical candidate can help predict the need for social support and physical rehabilitation services [2]. Functional assessment tools that have been validated in the elderly include the activities of daily living dependency score (ADL) and the instrumental activities of daily living dependency score (IADL) [2]. More recently a comprehensive multidisciplinary approach, the Comprehensive Geriatric Assessment (CGA), has proven effective in both risk stratifying patients prior to intervention and minimizing postoperative morbidity [2]. Consideration of CGA prior to surgical intervention improves functional status postoperatively and reduces hospital and nursing home stays, thereby decreasing overall medical costs [8].

Recent data show that 56% of newly diagnosed cancers and 71% of cancer deaths occur in individuals >65 years [9]. Multiple factors often need to be addressed when considering cancer treatment in the geriatric population. The goals of cancer treatment in the elderly include minimizing the impact of treatment on QOL and maximizing long-term functioning and independence. Both physiologic and cognitive changes associated with aging can impact the elderly patient's ability to receive standard oncologic therapies and also may increase the risk associated with various surgical and nonsurgical cancer treatments. Functional status, cognition, comorbidity, life expectancy, and risk of functional decline all must be considered in the elderly cancer patient [10]. Unfortunately few oncology clinical trials include significant numbers of elderly patients, rendering it difficult to extrapolate standard cancer therapy to this age group. Thus, pretreatment assessment of the elderly cancer patient's overall health status is imperative.

Prostate Cancer

Introduction

Prostate cancer is the most commonly diagnosed cancer in North American and European men [11]. Despite the significant worldwide burden of the disease, little is known about the etiology of prostate cancer. The incidence of prostate cancer increases with increasing age, documented both clinically and in autopsy studies [11]. The relationship between rising incidence of prostate cancer and age exists both in the U.S [12] and in Europe [13]. Analysis of recent Surveillance, Epidemiology, and End Results (SEER) data, revealed that the median age at diagnosis is 67 years with over 70% of prostate cancer deaths occurring in men older than 75 years. Indeed, over 20% of new prostate cancer diagnoses occur in men older than 75 years [14]. It is estimated that, by 2030, 20% of men in the U.S. will be older than 65 years, thereby underscoring the significant public health burden of prostate cancer diagnosis and treatment in the U.S. over the next two decades [15].

Assessment of Comorbidity and Relative Life Expectancy

Given the dramatic impact of PSA screening on prostate cancer diagnosis over the past 20 years, careful consideration must be paid to assessment of patient comorbidity, life expectancy, quality of life, and specific utility functions when deciding whom to screen for prostate cancer. As with any medical decision surrounding whether to treat or not treat an illness, the risk of disease must be balanced against risk of treatment both in terms of survival and health-related quality of life (HRQOL). Prostate cancer is no exception to this rule. The lengthy natural history of the disease and the advanced age at which the disease is frequently diagnosed have raised real questions regarding the need to diagnose (or treat) prostate cancer in patients of advanced age. Management of prostate cancer in the elderly affords clinicians the opportunity to commit two significant errors: "ageism," which refers to denying effective management to someone based strictly upon age as well as "overtreatment," which refers to the administration of toxic therapies to patients for diseases that, left untreated, are unlikely to result in significant morbidity or mortality [16]. The goal of prostate cancer management in the elderly is to withhold screening and treatment in those who are unlikely to benefit and to promote screening and treatment in those who are most likely to benefit.

A patient's remaining life expectancy (RLE) must to be incorporated into patient-specific decision-making. Additionally, one must estimate the likelihood that intervention such as screening or treatment would benefit the patient within the estimated RLE. Estimation of life expectancy is of utmost importance in an elderly prostate cancer population given the approximately 10-year lead time to associated morbidity and mortality from screen detected prostate cancers [17]. Careful attention to life-expectancy tables is helpful when considering prostate cancer treatment in the elderly. Walter and Covinsky evaluated life expectancy and risk of death from various solid tumors in both men and women. Evaluation of life-expectancy tables reveals that, for a healthy 75-year-old male (top 25th percentile), the patient is expected to live in excess of 14 years, however, for a relatively unhealthy male (bottom 25th percentile), the patient's life expectancy is a mere 4.9 years [18].

Assessment of comorbidity and competing risks permits estimation of overall health status and life expectancy. Unfortunately, current risk-stratification models cannot predict with complete accuracy those who would benefit from treatment and those who can safely be managed expectantly. Numerous groups have performed competing-risks analysis to determine the likelihood of prostate cancer death compared to death from other causes. Most recently Albertson et al. demonstrated that, for men older than 75-years with no comorbidity and intermediate-risk prostate cancer, the risk of all-cause mortality at 10 years is 67.1% compared to 14.0% for prostate cancer-specific mortality. Men with two or more comorbidities were found to have a risk of all-cause mortality of 74.4% compared to prostate cancer-specific mortality of 5.0% (Table 9.1) [19]. Numerous comorbidity indices have been studied in prostate cancer populations with particular attention to identifying those patients at significant risk of death from non-prostate cancer etiologies. Boulos et al. evaluated five comorbidity indices and found that the Chronic Disease Score (CDS), Index of Coexistent Disease (ICED), and the Cumulative Illness Rating Scale (CIRS) outperformed more commonly used methods such as the CCI in the population studied [20]. While clinicians frequently make casual judgment regarding the degree of overall health and patient comorbidity, judicious use of validated comorbidity indices may improve prediction of risk of both prostate cancer-specific and all-cause mortality and ultimately improve patient-specific decision-making. As discussed above, however, evaluation of comorbidity must be taken in the context of patient-specific disability, frailty, functional dependence, the presence or absence of geriatric syndromes, and vulnerability [16].

PSA Screening in the Elderly

Since the introduction and widespread implementation of PSA screening in the early 1990s there has been a significant prostate cancer stage migration, favoring the diagnosis of low-grade, low-stage disease [21]. This stage migration, coupled with the remarkable prevalence of histologic prostate cancer at autopsy, has prompted many clinicians and patients alike to question the necessity of PSA screening. Two recent randomized trials reported interim survival results detailing the effectiveness of PSA screening on both overall and prostate cancer-specific mortality. The Prostate, Lung, Colorectal, and Ovarian Cancer Screening Trial (PLCO) randomized 76,693 men to yearly prostate cancer screening with PSA and digital rectal examination (DRE) for 6 and 4 years, respectively. The risk of prostate cancer diagnosis was 116 per 10,000 person-years and 95 per 10,000 person-years in the screening and control groups, respectively. The risk of prostate cancer death was found to be 2.0 per 10,000 person-years and 1.7 per 10,000 person-years in the screening and control groups, respectively indicating both a very low rate of prostate cancer death and a lack of protection conferred by prostate cancer screening [22]. The PCLO study has been widely criticized due to the high rate of contamination found of the control group. Specifically, 52% of the patients randomized to the control arm of the study were screened with PSA testing by year 6, leading many to surmise that, while the survival benefit of PSA screening may indeed be small, this effect is largely attenuated by the high rate of screening in the control arm of the PLCO trial. The European Randomised Study of Screening for Prostate Cancer (ERSPC) randomized 182,000 men between the ages of 50 and 74 years to prostate cancer screening or no prostate cancer screening. Unlike the PLCO study, screening in the European randomized trial occurred, on average, every 4 years. The risk of prostate cancer diagnosis was found to be 8.2% and 4.8% in the screening and control arms, respectively. In the overall cohort, prostate cancer screening conferred a 20% reduction in the risk of prostate cancer-mortality. Excluding noncompliant study participants, the prostate cancer-specific mortality benefit improved to 27%. Despite these findings, investigators determined that 1,410 men would have to be screened and 48 men treated to prevent one prostate cancer death [23]. Despite the need to screen and treat a large number of men to prevent few prostate cancer deaths, many believe that longer follow-up will result in a larger observed survival benefit with PSA screening. Modeling the number needed to screen (NNS) and number needed to treat (NNT) in the ERSPC study reveals that, by 12 years of follow-up, the NNS and NNT will be 503 and 18, respectively [24].

What are the explanations for the disparate findings in the PLCO and ERSPC studies? Most point to two significant differences between the studies, namely vastly different rates of PSA screening/contamination of the control groups, and the variable rates of PSA "prescreening" amongst study participants. Indeed, nearly half of the patients assigned to the control arm of the PLCO study were subject to PSA screening during the trial likely leading to the modest increase in prostate cancer detection (17%) in the screening arm compared to the control arm. The rate of contamination of the ERSPC study was significantly less, and the incremental increase in prostate cancer detection in the screening arm was much higher than the PCLO study (71%). Additionally, half of the patients in the PLCO study underwent PSA testing and digital rectal exam (DRE) within 3 years of enrollment leading many to surmise that the prescreened nature of the control arm of the PCLO study attenuated any meaningful difference in prostate cancer-specific mortality [25].

Given the challenges in the interpretation of the recent randomized trials, not surprisingly, the appropriate use of PSA screening in older age males remains even less clear. Indeed, the risk of prostate cancer overdetection increases with increasing age with PSA testing resulting in an overdetection rate of 27% at 55 years and 56% by 75 years [17]. Nonetheless, the likelihood of high-risk prostate cancer increases with age accounting for 43% of tumors diagnosed in men older than 75 years as compared to 25% of tumors diagnosed in men younger than 75 years [26]. Assessment of individual comorbidity, family longevity, and overall health status in addition to ascertainment of patient-specific attitudes towards screening and treatment is necessary in order to allow patients to make well-informed decisions surrounding

Table 9.1 Overall and prostate cancer-specific mortality rates for men by years with localized prostate cancer (T1c)

Characteristic	Age at diagnosis							
	66–74 Years				75+ Years			
	5-Year mortality		10-Year mortality		5-Year mortality		10-Year mortality	
	Rate per 100[a]	95% CI[b]	Rate per 100[a]	95% CI[b]	Rate per 100[a]	95% CI[b]	Rate per 100[a]	95% CI[b]
T1c, Gleason 5–7, co morbidity = 0								
Overall mortality	11.7	10.2–13.1	28.8	25.3–32.6	26.3	24.8–28.0	67.1	63–72.4
Prostate cancer specific mortality	1.6	1.1–2.4	4.8	2.8–8.4	4.4	3.4–5.1	14.0	10.6–20.9
T1c, Gleason 5–7, co morbidity = 1								
Overall mortality	25.3	20.7–29.5	50.5	41.5–59.2	39.4	35.9–42.5	76.8	70.5–82.9
Prostate cancer-specific mortality	1.1	0.0–2.7	2.0	0.0–5.3	5.1	3.3–7.2	9.1	5.5–14.4
T1c, Gleason 5–7, co morbidity ≥2								
Overall mortality	42.5	36.1–48.5	83.1	67.4–97.2	48.1	42.7–52.7	74.4	63.7–84.7
Prostate cancer-specific mortality	4.3	1.6–8.3	5.3	2.5–10.0	4.0	1.7–6.5	5.0	2.5–8.7
T1c, Gleason 8–10, co morbidity = 0								
Overall mortality	26.4	22.2–30.8	55.0	43.9–65.9	41.4	38.3–44.0	77.0	71.5 to 82.5
Prostate cancer specific mortality	13.6	9.6–17.8	25.7	15.9–40.6	16.3	13.8–19.4	27.5	21.5 to 36.5

T1c, Gleason 8–10, comorbidity = 1								
Overall mortality	30.7	23.7–41.0	52.0	38.0–77.0	47.2	41.8–52.5	92.4	79.3 to 99.7
Prostate cancer-specific mortality	11.6	3.0–23.4	20.2	4.1–46.6	11.2	7.3–16.1	23.7	9.5 to 44.7
T1c, Gleason 8–10, comorbidity ≥2								
Overall mortality	52.0	42.1–64.5	64.3	52.0–84.9	65.7	55.9–70.1	94.3	87.4–100.0
Prostate cancer-specific mortality	9.6	2.4–19.3	13.7	2.7–33.4	12.8	7.3–18.9	18.8	9.3–36.8

[a]The mortality rates were derived by using smoothed cumulative incidence curves as described in the text
[b]CIs were estimated using a bootstrap with 1,000 replications

participation in PSA screening. While no consensus guidelines exist to direct physicians as to when to discontinue prostate cancer screening in older men, the U.S Preventative Services Task Force (USPSTF) has recommended discontinuing PSA screening in those patients older than 75 years of age [27–29]. Critics of the USPSTF guidelines argue that patients should be assessed for overall health based upon individual factors and not upon chronological age. Indeed, 78% of men surveyed at a prostate cancer screening clinic disagreed with the recommendation to discontinue screening at age 75 [30]. Given the limitations of the USPSTF recommendations, the most recent American Urological Association best practice statement advocates for an individualized approach to prostate cancer screening in patients of advanced age given the heterogeneity of overall health status amongst elderly patients [28]. Despite little evidence to support the benefit of PSA screening in elderly populations, the prevalence of screening in the USA population remains high [31]. In fact, some series indicate that the rate of screening is higher in those patients over age 70 than in those patients in their 50s [32]. Nonetheless, some evidence indicates that the rate of PSA testing among men older than 75 years declined after the publication of the U.S. Preventative Services Task Force recommendation and has continued to decline since the publication of the PLCO and ERSPC studies [33].

Considering the challenges imposed by PSA screening in the elderly, substantial effort has been directed at identifying very low-risk populations of elderly patients in whom PSA screening can be withheld. A recent longitudinal cohort study of men undergoing PSA screening revealed that no men between 75 and 80 years of age with a PSA of <3.0 ng/mL died of prostate cancer, potentially identifying a subset of men in which PSA screening could be safely omitted [34]. Additional similar identifying variables would benefit this and younger age groups.

Treatment of Localized Prostate Cancer

Most prostate cancers currently detected in the U.S. are clinically localized. Although many such men have low- or intermediate-risk disease, a significant majority seek active treatment [21]. Indeed, recent data suggests that 81.7% of men older than 75 receive active treatment for newly diagnosed prostate cancer. While a higher proportion of patients with high-risk disease receive active treatment (86.4%) when compared to those with low-risk disease (72.2%), this difference is modest [35]. The decision surrounding whether to undertake active treatment for localized prostate cancer in an older man must take into account the likelihood of death from prostate cancer, the risk of symptomatic metastatic disease, and the risk of death from other causes. Observational data suggests that elderly men do enjoy more favorable overall survival when treated for low- and intermediate-risk prostate cancer. Indeed, men 65–80 years old who underwent active treatment for prostate cancer were found to have a statistically significant survival advantage when compared to men that did not undergo active treatment (HR 0.69, 95% CI 0.66–0.72) even after controlling for comorbidity and other confounding variables [36].

While tools for the evaluation of comorbidity and assessment of overall health have been previously described, there are numerous risk-stratification schemes that aid in the prediction of outcome following treatment. Specifically, D'Amico et al. evaluated the risk of biochemical recurrence 5-years after definitive therapy for prostate cancer [37] and were able to stratify patients into low-, intermediate-, and high-risk subgroups based upon clinical stage, PSA, and Gleason Score. Within this risk-stratification scheme, low-risk patients are identified as having clinical stage T1c or T2a disease, PSA ≤10, and Gleason score ≤6. Intermediate-risk patients have clinical stage T2b disease, PSA >10 but ≤20, or Gleason score 7 disease, and finally high-risk patients were defined as clinical stage T2c or greater, PSA >20, or Gleason score ≥8. These risk-groups provide a framework upon which the clinician can assess global prostate cancer risk. In addition to D'Amico's widely utilized risk-stratification schema, there have been a number of published nomograms evaluating the risk of freedom from progression following radical prostatectomy [38], brachytherapy [39], and external beam radiation therapy (EBRT) [40]. Additionally, a model has been developed aids in the prediction of prostate cancer-specific survival following radical prostatectomy [41]. Combining these tools with previously described methods of assessment of comorbidity and overall health provides patient-specific information upon which to base treatment recommendations.

There are numerous well-described management options for a patient diagnosed with clinically organ confined prostate cancer including radical prostatectomy, external beam radiotherapy, brachytherapy, or active surveillance. Radical prostatectomy (RP) involves surgical removal of the prostate and seminal vesicles, and frequently involves staging pelvic lymphadenectomy. Historically this procedure was performed using an open surgical approach through a low-midline abdominal incision. More recently, robotic-assisted laparoscopic radical prostatectomy (RALP) has been popularized secondary to potential benefits with regard to improved blood loss and improved time to convalescence [42]. Advances in open surgical technique during the 1970s and 1980s resulted in significant improvements in the morbidity associated with RP. Specifically, attention to the dorsal venous complex resulted in a reduction in operative blood loss and novel nerve-sparing techniques improved functional outcomes such as continence and erectile function [43]. Despite these improvements, RP has generally not been performed in patients over age 70 due to concern regarding the risk of perioperative mortality in patients of advanced age. The AUA guidelines identify the patient most likely to benefit from RP as having a relatively long life expectancy, no significant surgical risk factors, and a preference for surgery [44, 45]. The European Association of Urology defines RP as standard treatment in patients with stage T1b-T2b, Nx-N0, M0 disease with a life expectancy greater than 10 years. The EAU defines RP as optional in younger patients with T1a disease and a long life expectancy and in patients with limited T3a disease, Gleason score 8 or less, PSA 20 ng/mL or less, and long life expectancy [45, 46].

Few series have evaluated functional outcomes from RP in the elderly. Kerr and Zeinke reviewed the Mayo clinic experience of 51 patients older than 75 years who underwent RP and found that two-thirds of elderly patients undergoing RP were without perioperative complication. Nonetheless, elderly patients were found to have a significantly higher rate of urinary incontinence following RP than their younger counterparts (16% vs. 3%) [47]. Data from Begg et al. support the finding that chronological age appears to directly impact the risk of urinary incontinence following radical prostatectomy. The risk of perioperative death, however, was found to more strongly associate with comorbidity than chronological age [48]. There are few data that specifically address functional outcomes in elderly men following RALP. Shikanov et al., in their single-institution series, found age to be independently associated with the risk of postoperative continence and potency [49].

While there are few randomized trials which compare treatments for clinically localized prostate cancer, there is randomized data that evaluates differences in prostate cancer-related death amongst patients undergoing radical prostatectomy compared to those randomized to watchful waiting. In the Scandinavian Prostate Cancer Group Study Number 4 (SPCG-4), 695 men with clinically localized prostate cancer were randomized to undergo radical prostatectomy or watchful waiting with initiation of androgen ablation in the context of disease progression. Radical prostatectomy resulted in a relative risk of prostate cancer-related death of 0.56 (95% CI 0.36–0.88) at 10 years [50] and 0.62 (0.44–0.87) at 12 years [51], corresponding to a NNT of 15. Those patients randomized to radical prostatectomy also enjoyed more favorable rates of distant metastases, local progression, and overall survival. Nonetheless, in the subgroup of patients older than 65 years there was no discernable difference in prostate cancer-specific mortality, overall mortality, or the risk of distant metastases [50, 51]. The authors do caution that the SPCG-4 study was not powered to detect small survival within subgroups, however these data call into question the routine recommendation of radical therapy for clinically localized prostate cancer in the elderly. The application of a "one size fits all" approach, however, is not advisable considering the remarkable heterogeneity of prostate cancer, and as described above, patient-specific risk of prostate cancer death must be balanced against death from other cases.

Indeed, while the SPCG-4 study failed to reveal any difference in prostate cancer-specific mortality amongst those patients older than 65 years treated with radical prostatectomy or watchful waiting, there is data to suggest that elderly patients with high-risk disease do benefit from the addition of external beam radiotherapy to androgen ablation. The SCPG-7/SFUO-3 study randomized patients with high-risk prostate cancer to receive androgen ablation or androgen ablation plus external beam radiotherapy. At a median of 10.8 years follow-up, those patients who received radiotherapy were found to have a relative risk of death from prostate cancer of 0.44 (95% CI 0.33–0.66). The magnitude of absolute risk reduction was higher in those patients older than 67 years when compared to those younger than 67 years (12.9% vs. 9.8%, respectively) [52]. It is clear that some patients stand to benefit from definitive therapy for prostate cancer and some patients do not. The most significant challenge in treating elderly patients with prostate cancer is determining whether an individual patient is part of the former group or the latter.

EBRT remains a mainstay of treatment for clinically localized prostate cancer in the elderly. The AUA guidelines identify the patient most likely to benefit from EBRT as having a relatively long life expectancy, no significant risk factors for radiation toxicity, and a preference for EBRT [44, 45]. Additionally, the EAU guidelines recommend that treatment decision should be based upon TNM classification, Gleason score, baseline PSA, age, comorbidity, life expectancy, and health-related quality of life (HRQOL). Specific recommendations include the use of 3D-conformal radiation therapy (CRT) with or without intensity modulated radiation therapy (IMRT) for patients with T1c-T2c N0 M0 disease with dose escalation for those patients with intermediate-risk disease (T2b, PSA 10–20, Gleason score 7) [45, 46].

The question of whether one should be treated for prostate cancer revolves largely around the patient's burden of comorbid disease and desire for treatment. Generally, the rates of biochemical control and cancer-specific survival are similar when comparing external beam radiotherapy and radical prostatectomy [53, 54]. As such, many practitioners who treat prostate cancer will base treatment recommendations upon a specific patient's utility function(s). As previously described, there has been a tendency amongst practitioners who treat prostate cancer to not recommend surgery in patients older than 70 years secondary to increasing risks of perioperative morbidity. External beam radiotherapy is feasible in patients of advanced age, however unlike radical prostatectomy, there are no randomized trials comparing radiation therapy to expectant management. Fiorica et al. recently evaluated their experience with radiotherapy for local and locally advanced prostate cancer in patients greater than 75 years. The authors determined that patients' burden of comorbid illness (as measured by the adult comorbidity evaluation index) was inversely related to overall survival. However, overall survival was not affected by receipt of EBRT. While comorbidity was found to strongly associate with the risk of acute bowel and urinary toxicity, there was no documented relationship between chronological age and acute or late toxicity [55]. This underscores the points raised previously in this chapter relating to the importance of careful assessment of patient comorbidity in the evaluation of both need for treatment and specific treatment choice. These data are consistent with previously published reports from pooled EORTC studies. Pignon et al. evaluated 1,619 patients who underwent radical radiotherapy for pelvic malignancy and determined that age was not associated with increasing radiation toxicity [56] thereby leading the investigators to conclude that chronologic age is not a limiting factor for radiotherapy for pelvic malignancy. These findings have been confirmed by a number of groups in a number of practice settings [57–59] leading many to conclude that radiotherapy is a reasonable treatment option for men with localized or locally advanced prostate cancer.

In addition to external beam radiotherapy, brachytherapy is a reasonable therapeutic option for men with localized low-risk disease. Unlike external beam radiation, brachytherapy is typically reserved for men with low-grade (Gleason score 6 or less) disease, minimal lower urinary tract symptoms, and small to moderate prostate volume (<50 g). In appropriately selected patients brachytherapy achieves excellent rates of biochemical progression-free survival, with cure rates approaching 99% in low-risk populations [60]. When compared to radical prostatectomy, patients undergoing brachytherapy tolerate the procedure quite well with favorable long-term quality of life outcomes [61]. Nonetheless, there are a number of problems with the general application of brachytherapy to the elderly population. Given the morbidity with regard to urinary function in men who undergo interstitial brachytherapy, many practitioners will not perform the procedure as primary prostate cancer treatment in men with significant pretreatment urinary bother (IPSS >15). Indeed, both pretreatment IPSS and prostate volume are strong predictors of posttreatment urinary toxicity in patients undergoing brachytherapy [62, 63]. Given the high prevalence of BPH and lower urinary tract symptoms in elderly men, there is considerable (and appropriate) concern over the long-term urinary morbidity of brachytherapy, which limits its general application. Furthermore, given the low-risk nature of most tumors treated by brachytherapy there is significant debate over whether or not any therapy (brachytherapy or otherwise) is indicated in elderly men with low-risk disease. Thus, while brachytherapy remains a treatment option for men with localized prostate cancer, it has not received wide acceptance in the elderly.

With the introduction and widespread dissemination of PSA screening in the early 1990s came a remarkable stage migration in prostate cancer epidemiology favoring the diagnosis of low-risk disease [21]. As discussed previously, this stage migration has generated a considerable amount of concern surrounding the overtreatment of clinically insignificant prostate tumors. Despite the nominal risk of prostate cancer-specific mortality in men diagnosed with low-risk disease, more than 90% of such men receive definitive treatment, typically in the form of surgery or radiation therapy [64]. Given the competing risks of overall mortality in the cohort of patients diagnosed with prostate cancer in contemporary series, there has been growing interest in active surveillance with curative intent, a paradigm by which patients are monitored until they demonstrate evidence of disease progression at which time definitive therapy is triggered. Active surveillance is dissimilar from watchful waiting, a paradigm by which patients are treated only should they develop symptoms often attributable to metastatic disease. Among the theoretical benefits of active surveillance is a significant reduction in prostate cancer overtreatment, particularly in elderly men who stand to benefit little from radical therapy.

Active surveillance series are beginning to mature, and while follow-up remains short- to intermediate-term, these series do show promising results. Enrollment criteria for the Johns Hopkins Active Surveillance program includes patients with clinical stage T1c disease, PSA density less than 0.15 ng/mL, Gleason score 6 or less, two or fewer biopsy cores with cancer, and a maximum of 50% involvement of any core with cancer [65]. The investigators have followed a total of 769 men with a median follow-up of 2.5 years and found that a total of 33% of men underwent intervention at a median time of 2.2 years with 73.7% of these men doing so for biopsy reclassification. Nonetheless, there were no men in the Johns Hopkins Program who developed distant metastatic disease or died from prostate cancer

[66]. Perhaps the most mature active surveillance cohort is from the University of Toronto, where the surveillance cohort is somewhat more heterogeneous. Enrollment criteria in the Toronto program currently include all low-risk patients (Gleason score 6 or less and PSA less than 10 ng/mL); however, from 1995 to 1999 the program did enroll patients older than 70 years with PSA up to 15 ng/mL or Gleason 3+4 disease. Investigators have followed 450 patients for a median of 6.8 years and reported a treatment rate of 30%. The 5- and 10-year cancer-specific survival in the cohort was 99.7% and 97.2%, respectively, with a hazard ratio for other-cause mortality of 18.6 (95% CI 7.6–45.7) [67].

While the risk of prostate cancer-specific mortality seems low compared to other competing causes of death, particularly in patients with a moderate to high burden of medical comorbidity, there remains some concern about missed opportunity for intervention. Warlick et al. evaluated the risk of "noncurable" cancer in patients undergoing immediate radical prostatectomy compared to delayed surgery after having been enrolled in an active surveillance program. Using a definition of "noncurable" cancer as adverse pathology associated with a less than 75% chance of remaining disease-free 10 years after surgery, the investigators found that, after adjustment for PSA density and age, there was no difference in the risk of "noncurable" cancer between those treated immediately and those undergoing delayed intervention [68]. This data indicates that there is little risk in enrollment in active surveillance with delayed intervention. There remains some controversy, however, regarding the safety of delayed treatment. O'Brien et al. evaluated patients with D'Amico low-risk disease and determined that those patients who suffered a treatment delay of 6 months or greater were found to have higher risk of pathologic upgrading and biochemical failure after prostatectomy. Surgical delay remained an independent predictor of biochemical failure on multivariable analysis when controlling for PSA and clinical stage [69]. Thus, while active surveillance appears to be a safe management strategy for many men with low-risk prostate cancer, long-term follow-up will be required to carefully assess the survival implications associated with delayed intervention. The elderly population, particularly elderly patients with low-risk disease, should certainly be counseled regarding the merits and pitfalls of active surveillance.

The diagnosis and management of elderly patients with prostate cancer remains a challenge to treating physicians. Unlike many other malignancies, the risk of diagnosis and treatment must be carefully considered in the context of competing risks of death. Working groups have begun to develop paradigms for prostate cancer management in the elderly. Utilization of prediction tools coupled with the use of such management paradigms (Fig. 9.1, [94]) will help clinicians and patients alike achieve optimal treatment strategies. While current prediction tools remain imperfect, they are helpful in the quantification of risk when counseling such patients. As data from ongoing studies begins to mature, we will continually have to reassess the paradigm of prostate cancer screening, diagnosis, and treatment.

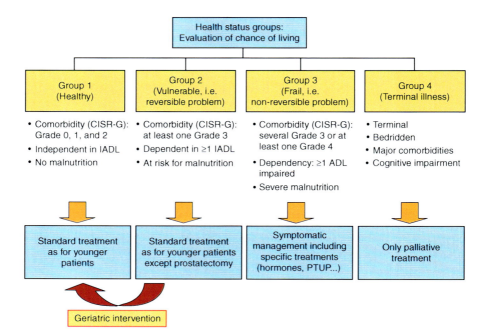

Fig. 9.1 A decision tree for treating patients with localized disease and metastatic disease

Bladder Cancer

Introduction and Epidemiology

Bladder cancer is a commonly diagnosed malignancy in both men and women, accounting for over 70,000 incident cases and over 14,000 deaths in 2010 [12]. Like many other malignancies, bladder cancer occurs most commonly in the elderly, with the median age at diagnosis being 69 and 71 years in men and women, respectively [70]. Indeed, the incidence of bladder cancer seems to increase with increasing age. Schultzel et al. evaluated the California Cancer Registry and determined that the incidence of bladder cancer peaks in those patients 85 years and older regardless of sex or ethnic background [71]. Interestingly, these investigators documented a 10 year difference in peak incidence between lung/bronchus cancer and bladder cancer despite similar risk factors such as smoking and occupational exposure [71]. Nonetheless, there is a strong association of bladder cancer incidence with age, with an overall incidence of 28.6% in patients under 65 years and 71.4% in those over 65 years [3].

Bladder cancer treatment and outcome is largely determined by disease grade and stage. While nonmuscle-invasive tumors are frequently managed with transurethral resection and intravesical immunotherapy/chemotherapy, muscle-invasive tumors require radical therapy traditionally in the form of radical cystectomy and urinary diversion. Given the significant difference in treatment strategy amongst patients with either nonmuscle-invasive or muscle-invasive disease, there is considerable interest in identifying relationships that exist between chronologic age and disease aggressiveness. Indeed, it seems as though there exists a direct relationship between age and the risk of diagnosis of muscle-invasive bladder cancer. Konety et al., using SEER data, found that the risk of muscle-invasive bladder cancer increases to 32.4% in those patients 85 years or older from 23.8% in those 55–64 years [72, 73]. This relationship was confirmed by Prout et al. who, using similar data, found the risk of muscle-invasive disease to be 28.7% in those patients 85 years or older compared to 19.4% in those less than 55 years [73, 74].

Nonmuscle-Invasive Bladder Cancer: Treatment Implications in the Elderly

As described above, the hallmarks of treatment for nonmuscle-invasive bladder cancer are transurethral resection and intravesical immunotherapy/chemotherapy. In the group of elderly patients with nonmuscle-invasive disease, endoscopic procedures including transurethral resection are generally well tolerated. Transurethral resection rarely creates scenarios in which major fluid shifts or pressures are transmitted to the cardiopulmonary, renal, or hepatic systems [3]. Generally, patients with low-grade, nonmuscle-invasive disease face little risk with regard to disease progression. Specifically, the risk of progression in patients with low-grade Ta disease is approximately 5–10% [75]. Emphasis is placed on local disease control, with particular attention paid to limiting the morbidity associated with such tumors. Patients with high-grade tumor(s), invasive disease, or carcinoma-in-situ, however, face higher risk of disease progression ranging from 15% to >50% [75] depending on the specific stage and grade of the tumor of interest. Traditionally, transurethral resection in combination with intravesical immunotherapy and/or chemotherapy has been used to reduce both disease recurrence and progression. Bacillus Calmette-Guerin (BCG) is the most common form of intravesical therapy used in the United States. Intravesical administration of BCG results in a local immune response with cytokine induction favoring interferon-γ and IL-2. Such response is thought to activate cell-mediated cytotoxic mechanisms that translate into disease control [75, 76].

The efficacy of intravesical BCG in reducing the likelihood of disease recurrence [75, 77–79] and progression [75, 80, 81] has been well described in the literature. Nonetheless, there is a growing body of evidence to suggest that the response to BCG is attenuated in the elderly. Joudi et al. evaluated data from a national phase II multicenter study of BCG plus interferon-alpha to assess differences in response to treatment based upon age. Investigators found the 2-year recurrence-free survival rates in patients 80 or older and 61–70 years to be 39% and 61%, respectively. The response rates [82] amongst elderly patients were lower than younger patients regardless of whether these patients were BCG-naïve or had been previously treated [83].

Herr reviewed the Memorial Sloan Kettering experience and found that, while there was no difference recurrence-free survival at 2 years, after 5 years, those patients older than 70 years demonstrated less favorable recurrence-free survival when compared to those younger than 70 years (27% vs. 37%, respectively) [84]. It is known that both innate and adaptive immunity declines with age [3, 85] and as such, it is theorized that elderly patients may not be able to mount the immune response necessary for optimal BCG response. Nonetheless, the magnitude of age as a negative predictor of response to intravesical BCG likely remains fairly small.

While the response to BCG appears to be somewhat attenuated with advancing age, there is some evidence to suggest that morbidity from treatment increases with advancing age. Heiner and Terris reviewed their experience of men receiving maintenance BCG and found the complication rate for patients less than 70 years and greater than 70 years to be 17.6% and 48.6%, respectively [86]. The most common complications reported in this series included cystitis/bladder pain severe enough to discontinue therapy, chills/fever, and severe prostatitis/epididymitis. These data led to the authors to conclude that maintenance should be given with caution in men over age 70 and should be avoided in patients over age 80 [86]. There are few other series that specifically address the risk of complication from intravesical BCG in the elderly; however, there are a number of case reports that raise concern over this association [82, 87, 88]. Clearly, the benefits of intravesical BCG with regard to reduction in the risk of disease recurrence and progression must be weighed against the risks of BCG therapy in patients of advanced age.

Muscle-Invasive Bladder Cancer: Treatment Implications in the Elderly

The gold standard treatment for muscle-invasive bladder cancer is radical cystectomy (RC) and urinary diversion [89]. Furthermore, recent data supports the use of neoadjuvant platinum-based chemotherapy in patients with muscle-invasive bladder cancer [90–92]. Nonetheless, radical surgery and systemic chemotherapy confer significant "stress" to a number of organ systems, and given the gradual decline in physiologic capacity among the elderly, each of these interventions is limited by the patients' abilities to tolerate the insult(s) of treatment [3]. Indeed, patients aged 75 years or older have, not surprisingly, a higher prevalence of cardiac disease prior cancer diagnosis, chronic anemia, and less favorable American Society of Anesthesiologists (ASA) Classification than those less than 75 years [74].

The substantial burden of comorbidity in patients of advanced age has resulted in dramatic variations in care amongst elderly patients with muscle-invasive bladder cancer. Prout et al., using SEER data, noted that patients over 80 years old were far less likely to receive RC than their younger counterparts (16% vs. 40–55%, respectively) [74]. These data were confirmed by Konety et al. who demonstrated that the risk of undergoing RC was lower in patients older than 75 years than patients younger than 75 years [72] and by Schrag et al. who demonstrated that patients older than 85 years had an adjusted odds ratio of undergoing cystectomy on 0.11 (95% CI 0.09–0.15) when compared to those 65–69 years old [93].

Hollenbeck et al. reported a cystectomy rate of 11.5% in those patients older than 80 years with muscle-invasive bladder cancer. Nonetheless, radical/partial cystectomy resulted in the greatest risk reduction in both bladder cancer-specific and overall mortality [94]. The exact nature of the bias for or against RC in the elderly is unknown, but possible reasons include delay in diagnosis, the inappropriate use of less aggressive therapy, or the perception that older patients would not tolerate a major operative procedure [4].

Variation in bladder cancer care amongst the elderly is not limited, however, to rates of surgical extirpation. Porter et al. evaluated the use of systemic chemotherapy for bladder cancer and demonstrated that age was indirectly associated with risk of receiving systemic chemotherapy [95]. With diminished functional reserve related to either advanced cancer or chronologic age, delivery of cytotoxic chemotherapy can prove particularly challenging in the elderly population [96]. Nonetheless, there are a number of questions as to why utilization of systemic chemotherapy in patients with muscle-invasive bladder cancer remains so poor. Certainly renal function compromise can result in reduced ability to administer chemotherapy, however, underutilization exists even in patients with acceptable renal function [97]. As with the variation in cystectomy rates, the reasons for such profound underutilization of systemic chemotherapy are likely multi-factorial. Nonetheless, more work must be done to identify barriers to improving the quality of care delivered to elderly patients with high-risk muscle-invasive bladder cancer.

Consideration of outcomes following RC in the elderly is challenging given the retrospective nature of many of the published case series, the varied definition of "elderly," and the failure amongst investigators to adequately evaluate comorbid disease and functional capacity. Indeed, the use of chronological age, as previously described, is far less informative than the careful assessment of comorbidity, functional capacity, and disability, particularly when considering major abdominal surgery in an elderly population. Chamie et al., using SEER data, demonstrated a survival advantage associated with RC in all age groups with the exception of octogenarians, who demonstrated only a 3 month overall survival benefit (18mo vs. 15mo) which improved when those with nodal or metastatic disease were excluded (23mo vs. 15mo) [98]. Fairey et al. found that chronological age was not associated with the risk of 90-day mortality or early postoperative complications, however, that comorbodity was a strong predictor of 90-day mortality and early postoperative complications [99]. Contrary to these findings, Liberman et al. demonstrated that both septuagenarian and octogenarian age increased the risk of 90-day mortality after RC [100]. Konety et al. found that increasing age was independently associated with in-hospital mortality after RC [101] and Hollenbeck et al. reported that increasing age was associated with increasing risk of postoperative complication after RC [102]. Koppie et al. incorporated age-adjusted Charlson comorbidity index (ACCI) into their evaluation of RC outcomes and determined that increasing ACCI was associated with increasing risk of pT3+ disease, decreasing likelihood of lymphadenectomy, and decreasing likelihood of postoperative chemotherapy. Furthermore, higher ACCI was associated with worse overall but similar recurrence-free survival [103]. Siegrist et al. evaluated the Memorial Sloan Kettering Experience and found that octogenarians experienced a nonsignificantly higher rate of minor (55% vs. 51%) and major (17% vs. 13%) complications compared to younger patients within 90 days of surgery, however, octogenarians were more likely to die within 90 days of surgery (6.8% vs. 2.2%, $p = 0.01$). Interestingly, while octogenarians were more likely to die of non-bladder cancer-related causes, bladder cancer-specific survival was similar between octogenarians and younger patients [104].

It is difficult to identify the reasons for differences between studies. While some series indicate that chronological age does afford some predictive value when it comes to the risk of complication or early mortality some fail to demonstrate this relationship. The decision to proceed with radical surgery should be individualized to allow for adequate consideration of chronologic age, comorbidity, and functional status. Doing so will permit the most comprehensive evaluation of individual risk and potential benefit from radical surgery. As RC has a demonstrable benefit in the geriatric population, chronologic age alone should not be used to exclude patients from surgery. In patients who are either unfit or unwilling to undergo RC, bladder sparing protocols in the form of systemic chemotherapy, external beam radiation, and aggressive transurethral resection may present a viable option [105]. However, bladder sparing protocols may be less likely to provide a cure, may adversely affect long-term quality of life, have significant side effects, and may only provide short-term palliation [106].

Noncontinent diversion in the form of an ileal conduit is the most common urinary diversion employed in elderly patients following RC [107]. Continent diversion in the form of an orthotopic neobladder or a cutaneous catheterizable reservoir offer the advantage of continence without the need for an external appliance, there is significant concern over the increased risk of complication in the elderly population [108, 109]. Furthermore, concerns have been raised over functional outcomes following continent diversion in the elderly. Madersbacher et al. evaluated functional outcomes following orthotopic neobladder and determined that increasing age was associated with lower reservoir capacity, increasing nocturia, and increasing rates of day and nighttime incontinence [110]. Hautmann et al. confirmed these findings, reporting an increased risk of incontinence in elderly patients undergoing orthotopic neobladder [110, 111]. Thus, the potential for improved quality of life and body image secondary to continent diversion must be balanced against the possibility of increased risk for perioperative complications and potentially adverse long-term functional outcomes.

Kidney Cancer

Introduction and Epidemiology

Renal cell carcinoma (RCC) remains a common malignancy among the elderly with over 58,000 new cases diagnosed in 2010 and over 13,000 deaths attributed to the disease during the same time period [12]. Furthermore, the incidence of RCC continues to rise in the United States with diagnosis rates of localized tumors outpacing that of advanced or metastatic disease [112, 113]. Many attribute the observed increase in diagnosis of localized RCC to the more liberal application of imaging techniques. Indeed, between 13 and 27% of abdominal imaging studies identify a renal lesion, the majority of which are benign cysts that require no treatment [114, 115]. Indeed, the largest increase in incidence of small renal masses has been observed in those patients older than 70 years, possibly owing to the frequent use of imaging in the elderly [116]. Whereas historically patients with RCC presented with the classic triad of hematuria, flank pain, and flank mass, in contemporary series the majority of new renal masses are diagnosed incidentally on imaging studies performed for non-renal indications [117, 118].

Kidney cancer is largely a disease of the elderly with the median age at diagnosis of 65 years with 25% of newly diagnosed patients older than 75 years [119]. As with other genitourinary malignancies, there are multiple considerations that must be taken into account when treating elderly patients with newly diagnosed RCC. There are conflicting data surrounding the implication(s) of age on clinicopathologic features at RCC diagnosis. Verhoest et al. evaluated 4,774 patients from various European centers and found that increasing age was associated with increasing tumor size and nuclear grade. Furthermore, increasing age was inversely associated with cancer-specific and overall survival [120]. Despite advances in cross-sectional imaging, nearly 20% of suspicious renal masses are benign at pathologic analysis [121]. Recent attention has been paid to active surveillance of small, incidentally detected renal masses. Kouba et al. observed 46 patients with small renal masses and found that the tumor growth rate was slower in patients over 60 years when compared to their younger counterparts (0.6 cm vs. 0.9 cm, respectively) [116]. Unfortunately, the relationship between age and RCC-specific outcome is poorly characterized and warrants further investigation.

As with other tumor types, considerable attention has been paid to the development of prognostic models for cancer-specific and overall mortality in attempt to define competing risks. These methods are particularly applicable in the elderly given the slow growth rate and low metastatic potential of small renal masses (<3 cm) [122]. Karakiewicz et al. recently developed a nomogram to predict 1, 2, 5, and 10-year RCC-specific survival. The model incorporates age, gender, the presence of symptoms, tumor size, T-stage, and the presence of metastatic disease and in an external validation cohort demonstrated excellent accuracy [123]. More recently, Kutikov et al., using a SEER cohort, found the overall risk of RCC-related death, other cancer death, and non-cancer death to be 4%, 7%, and 11%, respectively [124]. The investigators developed nomograms to predict the risk of death from RCC, risk of death from other cancer, and risk of non-cancer death which are particularly useful when counseling patients with a small renal mass and significant risk of perioperative morbidity. As with prostate and bladder cancer, it is critically important to incorporate validated prediction tools into everyday clinical practice. Doing so will allow patients to make informed, careful decisions about their care.

Treatment of Localized RCC in the Elderly

The last decade has brought significant change to the paradigm of treatment for localized RCC. Historically the gold standard of treatment for localized RCC was radical nephrectomy (RN) as described by Charles Robson [125]. However, growing concern over the risk of chronic kidney disease (CKD) secondary to radical nephrectomy has resulted in considerable interest in renal preservation in the form of nephron-sparing surgery (NSS), ablative techniques, and active surveillance (AS). Prior to undertaking any form of therapy for localized RCC careful attention must be paid to global renal function. Serum creatinine is not an accurate surrogate for overall renal function in the elderly, and as such, GFR should be estimated using a standardized equation such as the Modification of Diet in Renal Disease (MDRD) or performing a 24 h urine creatinine clearance [126]. Canter et al. evaluated the prevalence of baseline CKD in patients presenting to a referral cancer center with a solid renal tumor and found that 40% of patients 70 years or older had CKD stage III (GFR 30–60). Furthermore, 23% of patients older than 70 years had CKD stage III with a "normal" baseline serum creatinine (≤1.4 mg/dL) underscoring the need for GFR calculation in the elderly [127].

There is a well-documented relationship between CKD and the risk of death, cardiovascular events, and hospitalization [128, 129]. Furthermore, there is a growing body of evidence surrounding the incremental risk of CKD associated with undergoing radical nephrectomy when compared to partial nephrectomy. Huang et al. determined that patients undergoing RN were significantly more likely to suffer from stage III or greater CKD than those undergoing PN [130]. Furthermore, Thompson et al. evaluated the Mayo Clinic experience and identified patients treated with radical or partial nephrectomy for a solitary small renal mass and found that RN was associated with increased risk of death despite adjustment for known confounders and comorbidity [131] leading investigators to postulate that the observed increase in the risk of death may be attributed to increased risk of cardiovascular disease. Taken together, these data suggest that the risk of CKD following RN is significant, and given the known relationships between CKD and cardiovascular disease, efforts should be made to preserve renal function [132].

Surgical excision remains the gold standard for the treatment of localized RCC. While efforts should be made to preserve renal function, there remain circumstances in which NSS is not technically possible. As such, RN remains a therapeutic option for a patient with localized RCC in the most recent AUA guidelines [133]. Indeed, RN can be performed with acceptable morbidity in the elderly. Specifically, numerous series have evaluated the incremental morbidity associated with undergoing RN at advanced age and have not documented any increase in perioperative morbidity or mortality [134, 135]. There is increasing evidence that NSS affords patients comparable recurrence-free and long-term survival rates when compared to patients undergoing RN [132, 136]. Given the renal functional advantages afforded by NSS in the context of equivalent oncologic outcomes, the AUA guidelines do encourage physicians to counsel patients about the potential advantages of a nephron-sparing treatment approach in both the imperative and elective settings [133]. Furthermore, while historically NSS was performed for obligate indications, recent years have seen a profound expansion in utilization of NSS for larger, more complex, tumors. Longer follow-up will be required to determine whether the protective effects of renal preservation outweigh the potential oncologic risks incurred by these expanded indications.

In addition to surgical extirpation, there has been increasing interest in the use of ablative techniques in the treatment of localized RCC. Currently the two most common techniques include cryoablation and radiofrequency ablation (RFA). Either energy can be delivered percutaneously or laparoscopically. Given the relatively lower risk of major urological complication with the use of ablation when compared to open or laparoscopic partial nephrectomy [133] there has been considerable interest in applying this technique to elderly patients. Choueiri et al. found that, on multivariable adjusted analysis, age was directly associated with the risk of undergoing ablation for a small renal mass. The same study failed to demonstrate any difference in cancer-specific or overall survival between ablation and surgical extirpation [137]. Kunkle et al. performed a meta-analysis to evaluate the efficacy of various treatments for localized RCC and found that patients undergoing ablative techniques suffered from a higher risk of local recurrence, however, the investigators did not document any difference in metastatic progression [138]. Unfortunately, the comparative effectiveness data evaluating ablation and surgical extirpation is plagued by profound selection bias and short-term follow-up. Well-controlled prospective studies with long follow-up must be done to better characterize the role of ablation in the therapeutic armamentarium for localized RCC.

As described above, the widespread application of cross-sectional imaging has resulted in more frequent diagnosis of small, localized renal masses of uncertain clinical significance. Much like prostate cancer, the changing epidemiology of RCC has generated significant interest in active surveillance for small renal masses. Furthermore, analysis of population data has revealed increased rate of treatment for RCC, however, the death rate from the disease has paradoxically increased [139]. These data suggest that commonly treated small incidental renal tumors may be of little clinical significance and may not require active treatment. Indeed, numerous series have documented the relatively slow growth of small renal masses. Haramis et al. reviewed the Columbia University experience of patients with small renal masses subject to long-term follow-up and found the median growth rate to be 0.15 cm per year with only 4.5% of patients requiring delayed intervention. No patient in this series suffered from metastatic disease or cancer-related death. Other series have corroborated these data and have found that upwards of one-third of small renal masses demonstrate zero net growth at a median follow-up of 29 months [140]. Additionally, a recent meta-analysis determined that the risk of progression to metastatic disease was equivalent in patients undergoing active AS when compared to those undergoing extirpative surgery or ablative therapy [138]. Furthermore, retrospective data indicates that delayed intervention secondary to increase in tumor size does not portend any prognostic implication [141]. Taken together, these data suggest that AS is a reasonable treatment strategy for patients with small renal masses who are too debilitated to undergo active intervention or who are unwilling to accept the potential risks of such interventions.

Treatment of Metastatic Disease in the Elderly

One of the most salient questions in the management of elderly patients who present with metastatic disease is whether this group stands to benefit from cytoreductive nephrectomy. Overall survival for elderly patients who undergo cytoreductive nephrectomy in the setting of metastatic RCC has been shown to be similar to that of younger patients, albeit in a small sample size. However, cytoreductive nephrectomy is associated with an increased risk of perioperative mortality in those ≥75 years of age. Specifically, Kader et al. found the risk of perioperative mortality to be 21% in those older than 75 years and 1.1% in younger patients. The risk of a major operation in the setting of metastatic disease must be balanced with that of potential benefit on an individual basis in this age group [142].

Over the past decade numerous targeted systemic therapies have been approved for the treatment of metastatic RCC. While these therapies are not curative in the setting of advanced disease, treatment can provide improvement in progression-free survival; most commonly in patients with lower tumor burden and good performance status [143]. While there are few trials that specifically address comparative effectiveness of targeted therapy in the elderly, the available data does suggest that treatment efficacy is similar in older and younger populations. Subgroup analysis of the TARGET Study, a randomized trial evaluating the efficacy of sorafenib compared to placebo in patients who had been previously treated with systemic therapy demonstrated similar median progression-free survival amongst sorafenib-treated patients older and younger than 70 years. The risk of adverse events was similar amongst age groups, however, there was a slightly higher risk of grade 3 and 4 adverse events in the elderly (45.7% vs. 36.7%, respectively) [144]. Furthermore, in an Advanced RCC Sorafeib (ARCCS) expanded access program in which sorafenib was made available to patients not eligible for clinical trial, there was no observed difference in either response rates or adverse events between younger and older patients [145]. Phase III randomized data comparing sunitinib and interferon-alpha revealed no difference in clinical benefit and objective response rates between older and younger patients. Additionally, no differences in adverse events were identified between cohorts [146]. These data indicate that commonly used systemic therapies for metastatic RCC are safe and effective in the elderly. Longer follow-up and further investigation will be required to identify the optimal treatment paradigm for advanced disease in the elderly.

References

1. Etzioni DA, Liu JH, Maggard MA, Ko CY. The aging population and its impact on the surgery workforce. Ann Surg. 2003;238:170–7.
2. Pasetto LM, Lise M, Monfardini S. Preoperative assessment of elderly cancer patients. Crit Rev Oncol Hematol. 2007;64:10–8.
3. Shariat SF, Milowsky M, Droller MJ. Bladder cancer in the elderly. Urol Oncol. 2009;27:653–67.
4. Extermann M, Overcash J, Lyman GH, Parr J, Balducci L. Comorbidity and functional status are independent in older cancer patients. J Clin Oncol. 1998;16:1582–7.
5. Conwell Y, Forbes NT, Cox C, Caine ED. Validation of a measure of physical illness burden at autopsy: the cumulative illness rating scale. J Am Geriatr Soc. 1993;41:38–41.
6. Sanchez-Salas R, Prapotnich D, Rozet F, et al. Laparoscopic radical prostatectomy is feasible and effective in 'fit' senior men with localized prostate cancer. BJU Int. 2010;106:1530–6.
7. Guzzo TJ, Allaf ME, Pierorazio PM, et al. Perioperative outcomes of elderly patients undergoing laparoscopic renal procedures. Urology. 2009;73:572–6.
8. Rubenstein LZ, Stuck AE, Siu AL, Wieland D. Impacts of geriatric evaluation and management programs on defined outcomes: overview of the evidence. J Am Geriatr Soc. 1991;39:8S–16S; discussion 7S–8S.
9. SEER cancer statistics review. (1975–2002). National Cancer Institute. www.seer.cancer.gov/csr/1975_2002 Accessed Feb 2010.
10. Pal SK, Katheria V, Hurria A. Evaluating the older patient with cancer: understanding frailty and the geriatric assessment. CA Cancer J Clin. 2010;60:120–32.
11. Gronberg H. Prostate cancer epidemiology. Lancet. 2003;361:859–64.
12. Jemal A, Siegel R, Xu J, Ward E. Cancer statistics, 2010. CA Cancer J Clin. 2011;60:277–300.
13. Ferlay J, Autier P, Boniol M, Heanue M, Colombet M, Boyle P. Estimates of the cancer incidence and mortality in Europe in 2006. Ann Oncol. 2007;18:581–92.
14. Heinzer H, Steuber T. Prostate cancer in the elderly. Urol Oncol. 2009;27:668–72.
15. Crawford ED. Epidemiology of prostate cancer. Urology. 2003;62:3–12.
16. Mohile SG, Lachs M, Dale W. Management of prostate cancer in the older man. Semin Oncol. 2008;35:597–617.
17. Draisma G, Boer R, Otto SJ, et al. Lead times and overdetection due to prostate-specific antigen screening: estimates from the European Randomized Study of Screening for Prostate Cancer. J Natl Cancer Inst. 2003;95:868–78.
18. Walter LC, Covinsky KE. Cancer screening in elderly patients: a framework for individualized decision making. JAMA. 2001;285:2750–6.
19. Albertsen PC, Moore DF, Shih W, Lin Y, Li H, Lu-Yao GL. Impact of comorbidity on survival among men with localized prostate cancer. J Clin Oncol. 2011;29:1335–41.
20. Boulos DL, Groome PA, Brundage MD, et al. Predictive validity of five comorbidity indices in prostate carcinoma patients treated with curative intent. Cancer. 2006;106:1804–14.
21. Cooperberg MR, Lubeck DP, Meng MV, Mehta SS, Carroll PR. The changing face of low-risk prostate cancer: trends in clinical presentation and primary management. J Clin Oncol. 2004;22:2141–9.
22. Andriole GL, Crawford ED, Grubb 3rd RL, et al. Mortality results from a randomized prostate-cancer screening trial. N Engl J Med. 2009;360:1310–9.
23. Schroder FH, Hugosson J, Roobol MJ, et al. Screening and prostate-cancer mortality in a randomized European study. N Engl J Med. 2009;360:1320–8.
24. Loeb S, Vonesh EF, Metter EJ, Carter HB, Gann PH, Catalona WJ. What is the true number needed to screen and treat to save a life with prostate-specific antigen testing? J Clin Oncol. 2011;29:464–7.
25. Studer UE, Collette L. What can be concluded from the ERSPC and PLCO trial data? Urol Oncol. 2010;28:668–9.

26. Konety BR, Cowan JE, Carroll PR. Patterns of primary and secondary therapy for prostate cancer in elderly men: analysis of data from CaPSURE. J Urol. 2008;179:1797–803; discussion 803.
27. U.S. Preventive Services Task Force. Screening for prostate cancer: U.S. Preventive Services Task Force recommendation statement. Ann Intern Med. 2008;149:185–91.
28. Greene KL, Albertsen PC, Babaian RJ, et al. Prostate specific antigen best practice statement: 2009 update. J Urol. 2009;182:2232–41.
29. Smith RA, Cokkinides V, Brooks D, Saslow D, Brawley OW. Cancer screening in the United States, 2010: a review of current American Cancer Society guidelines and issues in cancer screening. CA Cancer J Clin. 2011;60:99–119.
30. Caire AA, Sun L, Robertson CN, et al. Public survey and survival data do not support recommendations to discontinue prostate-specific antigen screening in men at age 75. Urology. 2010;75:1122–7.
31. Walter LC, Bertenthal D, Lindquist K, Konety BR. PSA screening among elderly men with limited life expectancies. JAMA. 2006;296:2336–42.
32. Lu-Yao G, Stukel TA, Yao SL. Prostate-specific antigen screening in elderly men. J Natl Cancer Inst. 2003;95:1792–7.
33. Zeliadt SB, Hoffman RM, Etzioni R, Gore JL, Kessler LG, Lin DW. Influence of publication of US and European prostate cancer screening trials on PSA testing practices. J Natl Cancer Inst. 2010;103:520–3.
34. Schaeffer EM, Carter HB, Kettermann A, et al. Prostate specific antigen testing among the elderly—when to stop? J Urol. 2009;181:1606–14; discussion 13–4.
35. Roberts CB, Albertsen PC, Shao YH, et al. Patterns and correlates of prostate cancer treatment in older men. Am J Med. 2011;124:235–43.
36. Wong YN, Mitra N, Hudes G, et al. Survival associated with treatment vs observation of localized prostate cancer in elderly men. JAMA. 2006;296:2683–93.
37. D'Amico AV, Whittington R, Malkowicz SB, et al. Biochemical outcome after radical prostatectomy, external beam radiation therapy, or interstitial radiation therapy for clinically localized prostate cancer. JAMA. 1998;280:969–74.
38. Stephenson AJ, Scardino PT, Eastham JA, et al. Preoperative nomogram predicting the 10-year probability of prostate cancer recurrence after radical prostatectomy. J Natl Cancer Inst. 2006;98:715–7.
39. Kattan MW, Potters L, Blasko JC, et al. Pretreatment nomogram for predicting freedom from recurrence after permanent prostate brachytherapy in prostate cancer. Urology. 2001;58: 393–9.
40. Kattan MW, Zelefsky MJ, Kupelian PA, Scardino PT, Fuks Z, Leibel SA. Pretreatment nomogram for predicting the outcome of three-dimensional conformal radiotherapy in prostate cancer. J Clin Oncol. 2000;18:3352–9.
41. Stephenson AJ, Kattan MW, Eastham JA, et al. Prostate cancer-specific mortality after radical prostatectomy for patients treated in the prostate-specific antigen era. J Clin Oncol. 2009;27:4300–5.
42. Ficarra V, Cavalleri S, Novara G, Aragona M, Artibani W. Evidence from robot-assisted laparoscopic radical prostatectomy: a systematic review. Eur Urol. 2007;51:45–55; discussion 6.
43. Walsh PC. Anatomic radical prostatectomy: evolution of the surgical technique. J Urol. 1998;160:2418–24.
44. Thompson I, Thrasher JB, Aus G, et al. Guideline for the management of clinically localized prostate cancer: 2007 update. J Urol. 2007;177:2106–31.
45. Droz JP, Balducci L, Bolla M, et al. Management of prostate cancer in older men: recommendations of a working group of the International Society of Geriatric Oncology. BJU Int. 2010;106:462–9.
46. Heidenreich A, Aus G, Bolla M, et al. EAU guidelines on prostate cancer. Eur Urol. 2008;53:68–80.
47. Kerr LA, Zincke H. Radical retropubic prostatectomy for prostate cancer in the elderly and the young: complications and prognosis. Eur Urol. 1994;25:305–11; discussion 11–2.

48. Begg CB, Riedel ER, Bach PB, et al. Variations in morbidity after radical prostatectomy. N Engl J Med. 2002;346:1138–44.
49. Shikanov S, Desai V, Razmaria A, Zagaja GP, Shalhav AL. Robotic radical prostatectomy for elderly patients: probability of achieving continence and potency 1 year after surgery. J Urol. 2010;183:1803–7.
50. Bill-Axelson A, Holmberg L, Ruutu M, Garmo H, Stark JR, Busch C, Scandinavan Prostate Cancer Group Study No. 4, et al. Radical prostatectomy versus watchful waiting in early prostate cancer. N Engl J Med. 2005;352:1977–84.
51. Bill-Axelson A, Holmberg L, Ruutu M, Haggman M, Andersson SO, Bratell S, SPCG-4 Investigators, et al. Radical prostatectomy versus watchful waiting in early prostate cancer. N Engl J Med. 2011;364:1708–17.
52. Widmark A, Klepp O, Solberg A, et al. Endocrine treatment, with or without radiotherapy, in locally advanced prostate cancer (SPCG-7/SFUO-3): an open randomised phase III trial. Lancet. 2009;373:301–8.
53. Kupelian PA, Elshaikh M, Reddy CA, Zippe C, Klein EA. Comparison of the efficacy of local therapies for localized prostate cancer in the prostate-specific antigen era: a large single-institution experience with radical prostatectomy and external-beam radiotherapy. J Clin Oncol. 2002;20:3376–85.
54. Speight JL, Roach 3rd M. Radiotherapy in the management of clinically localized prostate cancer: evolving standards, consensus, controversies and new directions. J Clin Oncol. 2005;23:8176–85.
55. Fiorica F, Berretta M, Colosimo C, et al. Safety and efficacy of radiotherapy treatment in elderly patients with localized prostate cancer: a retrospective analysis. Arch Gerontol Geriatr. 2010;51:277–82.
56. Pignon T, Horiot JC, Bolla M, et al. Age is not a limiting factor for radical radiotherapy in pelvic malignancies. Radiother Oncol. 1997;42:107–20.
57. Nguyen TD, Azria D, Brochon D, et al. Curative external beam radiotherapy in patients over 80 years of age with localized prostate cancer: a retrospective rare cancer network study. Crit Rev Oncol Hematol. 2011;74:66–71.
58. Villa S, Bedini N, Fallai C, Olmi P. External beam radiotherapy in elderly patients with clinically localized prostate adenocarcinoma: age is not a problem. Crit Rev Oncol Hematol. 2003;48:215–25.
59. Ogawa K, Nakamura K, Onishi H, et al. Influence of age on the pattern and outcome of external beam radiotherapy for clinically localized prostate cancer. Anticancer Res. 2006;26:1319–25.
60. Taira AV, Merrick GS, Butler WM, et al. Long-term outcome for clinically localized prostate cancer treated with permanent interstitial brachytherapy. Int J Radiat Oncol Biol Phys. 2010;79:1336–42.
61. Crook JM, Gomez-Iturriaga A, Wallace K, et al. Comparison of health-related quality of life 5 years after SPIRIT: surgical prostatectomy versus interstitial radiation intervention trial. J Clin Oncol. 2011;29:362–8.
62. Roeloffzen EM, Vulpen MV, Battermann JJ, van Roermund JG, Saibishkumar EP, Monninkhof EM. Pretreatment nomogram to predict the risk of acute urinary retention after I-125 prostate brachytherapy. Int J Radiat Oncol Biol Phys. 2011;81:737–44.
63. Keyes M, Miller S, Moravan V, et al. Predictive factors for acute and late urinary toxicity after permanent prostate brachytherapy: long-term outcome in 712 consecutive patients. Int J Radiat Oncol Biol Phys. 2009;73:1023–32.
64. Cooperberg MR, Broering JM, Carroll PR. Time trends and local variation in primary treatment of localized prostate cancer. J Clin Oncol. 2011;28:1117–23.
65. Epstein JI, Walsh PC, Carmichael M, Brendler CB. Pathologic and clinical findings to predict tumor extent of nonpalpable (stage T1c) prostate cancer. JAMA. 1994;271:368–74.
66. Tosoian JJ, Trock BJ, Landis P, et al. Active surveillance program for prostate cancer: an update of the Johns Hopkins experience. J Clin Oncol. 2011;29:2185–90.
67. Klotz L, Zhang L, Lam A, Nam R, Mamedov A, Loblaw A. Clinical results of long-term follow-up of a large, active surveillance cohort with localized prostate cancer. J Clin Oncol. 2010;28:126–31.

68. Warlick C, Trock BJ, Landis P, Epstein JI, Carter HB. Delayed versus immediate surgical intervention and prostate cancer outcome. J Natl Cancer Inst. 2006;98:355–7.
69. O'Brien D, Loeb S, Carvalhal GF, et al. Delay of surgery in men with low risk prostate cancer. J Urol. 2010;185:2143–7.
70. Lynch CF, Cohen MB. Urinary system. Cancer. 1995;75:316–29.
71. Schultzel M, Saltzstein SL, Downs TM, Shimasaki S, Sanders C, Sadler GR. Late age (85 years or older) peak incidence of bladder cancer. J Urol. 2008;179:1302–5; discussion 5–6.
72. Konety BR, Joslyn SA. Factors influencing aggressive therapy for bladder cancer: an analysis of data from the SEER program. J Urol. 2003;170:1765–71.
73. Taylor 3rd JA, Kuchel GA. Bladder cancer in the elderly: clinical outcomes, basic mechanisms, and future research direction. Nat Clin Pract Urol. 2009;6:135–44.
74. Prout Jr GR, Wesley MN, Yancik R, Ries LA, Havlik RJ, Edwards BK. Age and comorbidity impact surgical therapy in older bladder carcinoma patients: a population-based study. Cancer. 2005;104:1638–47.
75. Jones JS, Campbell SC. Non-muscle-invasive bladder cancer. In: Wein AJ, editor. Campbell-Walsh urology. 9th ed. Philadelphia: Saunders Elsevier; 2007. p. 2448–67.
76. Bohle A, Brandau S. Immune mechanisms in bacillus Calmette-Guerin immunotherapy for superficial bladder cancer. J Urol. 2003;170:964–9.
77. Cookson MS, Sarosdy MF. Management of stage T1 superficial bladder cancer with intravesical bacillus Calmette-Guerin therapy. J Urol. 1992;148:797–801.
78. Jimenez-Cruz JF, Vera-Donoso CD, Leiva O, et al. Intravesical immunoprophylaxis in recurrent superficial bladder cancer (Stage T1): multicenter trial comparing bacille Calmette-Guerin and interferon-alpha. Urology. 1997;50:529–35.
79. Hurle R, Losa A, Ranieri A, Graziotti P, Lembo A. Low dose Pasteur bacillus Calmette-Guerin regimen in stage T1, grade 3 bladder cancer therapy. J Urol. 1996;156:1602–5.
80. Sylvester RJ, van der Meijden AP, Lamm DL. Intravesical bacillus Calmette-Guerin reduces the risk of progression in patients with superficial bladder cancer: a meta-analysis of the published results of randomized clinical trials. J Urol. 2002;168:1964–70.
81. Lamm DL, Blumenstein BA, Crissman JD, et al. Maintenance bacillus Calmette-Guerin immunotherapy for recurrent TA, T1 and carcinoma in situ transitional cell carcinoma of the bladder: a randomized Southwest Oncology Group Study. J Urol. 2000;163:1124–9.
82. Marans HY, Bekirov HM. Granulomatous hepatitis following intravesical bacillus Calmette-Guerin therapy for bladder carcinoma. J Urol. 1987;137:111–2.
83. Joudi FN, Smith BJ, O'Donnell MA, Konety BR. The impact of age on the response of patients with superficial bladder cancer to intravesical immunotherapy. J Urol. 2006;175:1634–9; discussion 9–40.
84. Herr HW. Age and outcome of superficial bladder cancer treated with bacille Calmette-Guerin therapy. Urology. 2007;70:65–8.
85. Solana R, Pawelec G, Tarazona R. Aging and innate immunity. Immunity. 2006;24:491–4.
86. Heiner JG, Terris MK. Effect of advanced age on the development of complications from intravesical bacillus Calmette-Guerin therapy. Urol Oncol. 2008;26:137–40.
87. Rawls WH, Lamm DL, Lowe BA, et al. Fatal sepsis following intravesical bacillus Calmette-Guerin administration for bladder cancer. J Urol. 1990;144:1328–30.
88. Gonzalez JA, Marcol BR, Wolf MC. Complications of intravesical bacillus Calmette-Guerin: a case report. J Urol. 1992;148:1892–3.
89. Huang GJ, Stein JP. Open radical cystectomy with lymphadenectomy remains the treatment of choice for invasive bladder cancer. Curr Opin Urol. 2007;17:369–75.
90. Grossman HB, Natale RB, Tangen CM, et al. Neoadjuvant chemotherapy plus cystectomy compared with cystectomy alone for locally advanced bladder cancer. N Engl J Med. 2003;349:859–66.
91. von der Maase H, Sengelov L, Roberts JT, et al. Long-term survival results of a randomized trial comparing gemcitabine plus cisplatin, with methotrexate, vinblastine, doxorubicin, plus cisplatin in patients with bladder cancer. J Clin Oncol. 2005;23:4602–8.

92. Advanced Bladder Cancer (ABC) Meta-analysis Collaboration. Neoadjuvant chemotherapy in invasive bladder cancer: update of a systematic review and meta-analysis of individual patient data advanced bladder cancer (ABC) meta-analysis collaboration. Eur Urol. 2005;48:202–5; discussion 5–6.
93. Schrag D, Mitra N, Xu F, et al. Cystectomy for muscle-invasive bladder cancer: patterns and outcomes of care in the Medicare population. Urology. 2005;65:1118–25.
94. Hollenbeck BK, Miller DC, Taub D, et al. Aggressive treatment for bladder cancer is associated with improved overall survival among patients 80 years old or older. Urology. 2004;64:292–7.
95. Porter MP, Kerrigan MC, Donato BM, Ramsey SD. Patterns of use of systemic chemotherapy for Medicare beneficiaries with urothelial bladder cancer. Urol Oncol. 2011;29:252–8.
96. Carreca I, Balducci L. Cancer chemotherapy in the older cancer patient. Urol Oncol. 2009;27:633–42.
97. Raj GV, Karavadia S, Schlomer B, et al. Contemporary use of perioperative cisplatin-based chemotherapy in patients with muscle-invasive bladder cancer. Cancer. 2010;117:276–82.
98. Chamie K, Hu B, Devere White RW, Ellison LM. Cystectomy in the elderly: does the survival benefit in younger patients translate to the octogenarians? BJU Int. 2008;102:284–90.
99. Fairey A, Chetner M, Metcalfe J, et al. Associations among age, comorbidity and clinical outcomes after radical cystectomy: results from the Alberta Urology Institute radical cystectomy database. J Urol. 2008;180:128–34; discussion 34.
100. Liberman D, Lughezzani G, Sun M, et al. Perioperative mortality is significantly greater in septuagenarian and octogenarian patients treated with radical cystectomy for urothelial carcinoma of the bladder. Urology. 2011;77:660–6.
101. Konety BR, Dhawan V, Allareddy V, Joslyn SA. Impact of hospital and surgeon volume on in-hospital mortality from radical cystectomy: data from the health care utilization project. J Urol. 2005;173:1695–700.
102. Hollenbeck BK, Miller DC, Taub D, et al. Identifying risk factors for potentially avoidable complications following radical cystectomy. J Urol. 2005;174:1231–7; discussion 7.
103. Koppie TM, Serio AM, Vickers AJ, et al. Age-adjusted Charlson comorbidity score is associated with treatment decisions and clinical outcomes for patients undergoing radical cystectomy for bladder cancer. Cancer. 2008;112:2384–92.
104. Donat SM, Siegrist T, Cronin A, Savage C, Milowsky MI, Herr HW. Radical cystectomy in octogenarians–does morbidity outweigh the potential survival benefits? J Urol. 2011;183:2171–7.
105. Tran E, Souhami L, Tanguay S, Rajan R. Bladder conservation treatment in the elderly population: results and prognostic factors of muscle-invasive bladder cancer. Am J Clin Oncol. 2009;32:333–7.
106. Montie JE. Against bladder sparing: surgery. J Urol. 1999;162:452–5; discussion 5–7.
107. Gore JL, Litwin MS. Quality of care in bladder cancer: trends in urinary diversion following radical cystectomy. World J Urol. 2009;27:45–50.
108. Sogni F, Brausi M, Frea B, et al. Morbidity and quality of life in elderly patients receiving ileal conduit or orthotopic neobladder after radical cystectomy for invasive bladder cancer. Urology. 2008;71:919–23.
109. Froehner M, Brausi MA, Herr HW, Muto G, Studer UE. Complications following radical cystectomy for bladder cancer in the elderly. Eur Urol. 2009;56:443–54.
110. Madersbacher S, Mohrle K, Burkhard F, Studer UE. Long-term voiding pattern of patients with ileal orthotopic bladder substitutes. J Urol. 2002;167:2052–7.
111. Hautmann RE, Miller K, Steiner U, Wenderoth U. The ileal neobladder: 6 years of experience with more than 200 patients. J Urol. 1993;150:40–5.
112. Chow WH, Dong LM, Devesa SS. Epidemiology and risk factors for kidney cancer. Nat Rev Urol. 2010;7:245–57.
113. Kane CJ, Mallin K, Ritchey J, Cooperberg MR, Carroll PR. Renal cell cancer stage migration: analysis of the National Cancer Data Base. Cancer. 2008;113:78–83.

114. Tada S, Yamagishi J, Kobayashi H, Hata Y, Kobari T. The incidence of simple renal cyst by computed tomography. Clin Radiol. 1983;34:437–9.
115. Hara AK, Johnson CD, MacCarty RL, Welch TJ. Incidental extracolonic findings at CT colonography. Radiology. 2000;215:353–7.
116. Kouba E, Smith A, McRackan D, Wallen EM, Pruthi RS. Watchful waiting for solid renal masses: insight into the natural history and results of delayed intervention. J Urol. 2007;177:466–70; discussion 70.
117. Jayson M, Sanders H. Increased incidence of serendipitously discovered renal cell carcinoma. Urology. 1998;51:203–5.
118. Luciani LG, Cestari R, Tallarigo C. Incidental renal cell carcinoma-age and stage characterization and clinical implications: study of 1092 patients (1982–1997). Urology. 2000;56:58–62.
119. Edwards BK, Brown ML, Wingo PA, et al. Annual report to the nation on the status of cancer, 1975–2002, featuring population-based trends in cancer treatment. J Natl Cancer Inst. 2005;97:1407–27.
120. Verhoest G, Veillard D, Guille F, et al. Relationship between age at diagnosis and clinicopathologic features of renal cell carcinoma. Eur Urol. 2007;51:1298–304; discussion 304–5.
121. Kutikov A, Fossett LK, Ramchandani P, et al. Incidence of benign pathologic findings at partial nephrectomy for solitary renal mass presumed to be renal cell carcinoma on preoperative imaging. Urology. 2006;68:737–40.
122. Chen DY, Uzzo RG. Optimal management of localized renal cell carcinoma: surgery, ablation, or active surveillance. J Natl Compr Canc Netw. 2009;7:635–42; quiz 43.
123. Karakiewicz PI, Suardi N, Capitanio U, et al. A preoperative prognostic model for patients treated with nephrectomy for renal cell carcinoma. Eur Urol. 2009;55:287–95.
124. Kutikov A, Egleston BL, Wong YN, Uzzo RG. Evaluating overall survival and competing risks of death in patients with localized renal cell carcinoma using a comprehensive nomogram. J Clin Oncol. 2011;28:311–7.
125. Robson CJ, Churchill BM, Anderson W. The results of radical nephrectomy for renal cell carcinoma. J Urol. 1969;101:297–301.
126. Carnevale V, Pastore L, Camaioni M, et al. Estimate of renal function in oldest old inpatients by MDRD study equation, Mayo Clinic equation and creatinine clearance. J Nephrol. 2010;23:306–13.
127. Canter D, Kutikov A, Sirohi M, et al. Prevalence of baseline chronic kidney disease in patients presenting with solid renal tumors. Urology. 2010;77:781–5.
128. Go AS, Chertow GM, Fan D, McCulloch CE, Hsu CY. Chronic kidney disease and the risks of death, cardiovascular events, and hospitalization. N Engl J Med. 2004;351:1296–305.
129. Foley RN, Wang C, Collins AJ. Cardiovascular risk factor profiles and kidney function stage in the US general population: the NHANES III study. Mayo Clin Proc. 2005;80:1270–7.
130. Huang WC, Levey AS, Serio AM, et al. Chronic kidney disease after nephrectomy in patients with renal cortical tumours: a retrospective cohort study. Lancet Oncol. 2006;7:735–40.
131. Thompson RH, Boorjian SA, Lohse CM, et al. Radical nephrectomy for pT1a renal masses may be associated with decreased overall survival compared with partial nephrectomy. J Urol. 2008;179:468–71; discussion 72–3.
132. Russo P. Partial nephrectomy for renal cancer: part I. BJU Int. 2011;105:1206–20.
133. Campbell SC, Novick AC, Belldegrun A, et al. Guideline for management of the clinical T1 renal mass. J Urol. 2009;182:1271–9.
134. Varkarakis I, Neururer R, Harabayashi T, Bartsch G, Peschel R. Laparoscopic radical nephrectomy in the elderly. BJU Int. 2004;94:517–20.
135. Pareek G, Yates J, Hedican S, Moon T, Nakada S. Laparoscopic renal surgery in the octogenarian. BJU Int. 2008;101:867–70.
136. Uzzo RG, Novick AC. Nephron sparing surgery for renal tumors: indications, techniques and outcomes. J Urol. 2001;166:6–18.
137. Choueiri TK, Schutz FA, Hevelone ND, et al. Thermal ablation vs surgery for localized kidney cancer: a surveillance, epidemiology, and end results (SEER) database analysis. Urology. 2011;78:93–8.

138. Kunkle DA, Egleston BL, Uzzo RG. Excise, ablate or observe: the small renal mass dilemma—a meta-analysis and review. J Urol. 2008;179:1227–33; discussion 33–4.
139. Hollingsworth JM, Miller DC, Daignault S, Hollenbeck BK. Rising incidence of small renal masses: a need to reassess treatment effect. J Natl Cancer Inst. 2006;98:1331–4.
140. Kunkle DA, Crispen PL, Chen DY, Greenberg RE, Uzzo RG. Enhancing renal masses with zero net growth during active surveillance. J Urol. 2007;177:849–53; discussion 53–4.
141. Crispen PL, Viterbo R, Fox EB, Greenberg RE, Chen DY, Uzzo RG. Delayed intervention of sporadic renal masses undergoing active surveillance. Cancer. 2008;112:1051–7.
142. Kader AK, Tamboli P, Luongo T, et al. Cytoreductive nephrectomy in the elderly patient: the M. D. Anderson Cancer Center experience. J Urol. 2007;177:855–60; discussion 60–1.
143. Bellmunt J, Negrier S, Escudier B, Awada A, Aapro M. The medical treatment of metastatic renal cell cancer in the elderly: position paper of a SIOG Taskforce. Crit Rev Oncol Hematol. 2009;69:64–72.
144. Eisen T, Oudard S, Szczylik C, et al. Sorafenib for older patients with renal cell carcinoma: subset analysis from a randomized trial. J Natl Cancer Inst. 2008;100:1454–63.
145. Bukowski RM, Stadler WM, McDermott DF, et al. Safety and efficacy of sorafenib in elderly patients treated in the North American advanced renal cell carcinoma sorafenib expanded access program. Oncology. 2010;78:340–7.
146. Motzer RJ, Hutson TE, Tomczak P, et al. Sunitinib versus interferon alfa in metastatic renal-cell carcinoma. N Engl J Med. 2007;356:115–24.

Chapter 10
Lower Urinary Tract Symptoms

Ariana L. Smith and Alan J. Wein

Introduction

The lower urinary tract consists of interrelated structures including the bladder, urethra, smooth, and striated sphincters, pelvic floor muscles, and the prostate gland in men with a common function of providing effective urinary storage and voluntary urinary expulsion. These functions are achieved in two discrete phases of micturition [1].

Phase one involves filling and storage of urine in the bladder and is accomplished through:

1. Accommodation of increasing volumes of urine at low intravesical pressure
2. Appropriate sensation of bladder filling without allodynia
3. A bladder outlet that is closed at rest remains closed despite increases in intra-abdominal pressure
4. The absence of involuntary detrusor contractions (IVCs)

Phase two involves voiding and complete emptying of the bladder and is accomplished through:

1. Coordinated contraction of the bladder smooth muscle with adequate, magnitude and duration

A.L. Smith
Department of Urology, Hospital of the University of Pennsylvania and Pennsylvania Hospital, Philadelphia, PA 19106, USA

A.J. Wein (✉)
Division of Urology, Perelman Center for Advanced Medicine,
Hospital of the University of Pennsylvania, Philadelphia, PA 19104, USA
e-mail: alan.wein@uphs.upenn.edu

T.J. Guzzo et al. (eds.), *Primer of Geriatric Urology*, DOI 10.1007/978-1-4614-4773-3_10,   125
© Springer Science+Business Media New York 2013

Table 10.1 Lower urinary tract symptoms

Obstructive symptoms	Overactive symptoms	Incontinence symptoms
Hesitancy	Frequency	Urinary incontinence
Decreased force of stream	Nocturia	Stress incontinence
Intermittency	Urgency	Urgency incontinence
Straining	Urgency incontinence	Mixed incontinence
Position-dependent micturition	Increased sensation	Postural incontinence
Incomplete emptying	Dysuria	Nocturnal enuresis
Double voiding	Bladder pain	Continuous incontinence
Post void dribbling		Insensible incontinence
Urinary retention		Coital incontinence

2. Concomitant lowering of resistance at the level of the smooth and striated, urethral sphincter
3. The absence of anatomic obstruction

During normal physiologic filling, bladder sensation is nearly imperceptible and inhibitory reflexes prevent bladder contraction while the guarding reflex increases striated sphincter activity. At or near capacity the sensation of bladder fullness is responsible for initiating voluntary emptying of the bladder. Coordinated contraction of the bladder smooth muscle and relaxation of the urethral smooth and striated muscle leads to decreased outlet resistance, funneling of the bladder outlet, and facilitates complete bladder emptying. In the healthy adult, the facilitory and inhibitory neurologic impulses that regulate these processes are under full conscious control [2].

Lower urinary tract dysfunction is a term that has replaced voiding dysfunction as a descriptor of a broad category of abnormalities resulting from disruption of any one of the factors listed above; essentially a failure store, a failure to empty, or any combination of these factors. Lower urinary tract dysfunction can result in what has been termed *lower urinary tract symptoms*, or LUTS [3]. The term "prostatism", previously used to refer to male urinary tract symptoms of any cause, has been abandoned due to confusion over the causal relationship between these symptoms and the prostate.

Several age-related changes in lower urinary tract function can develop, producing at times bothersome LUTS. Prostatic growth increases with age in men and may lead to benign prostatic enlargement (BPE) with patients complaining of hesitancy, decreased force of urinary stream, incomplete bladder emptying, and at times frank urinary retention. The diagnosis of overactive bladder (OAB) increases with age in both men and women and consists of symptoms such as urgency, urinary frequency, nocturia, and urgency urinary incontinence (UUI) [4]. Other types of urinary incontinence are also common in the geriatric population; these include stress urinary incontinence (SUI), overflow incontinence, and mixed urinary incontinence.

A variety of symptoms as well as a variety of classification schemes for these symptoms exists. The most popular divides LUTS into filling/storage symptoms and voiding/emptying symptoms. For purposes of this chapter however, symptoms will be classified into three broad categories: (1) LUTS suggestive of obstruction, (2) LUTS suggestive of OAB, and (3) Urinary Incontinence (Table 10.1). Many patients, however, present with a combination of symptoms coming from more than one of these categories [5].

LUTS Suggestive of Obstruction

LUTS suggestive of obstruction occur during the voiding/emptying phase of micturition or immediately following. Patients may experience one or a multitude of urinary symptoms of varying severities. Patients tend to seek care when symptoms become bothersome, interrupt sleep, or lead to embarrassment.

Symptoms suggestive of obstruction are described below [6].

Urinary *hesitancy* is the complaint of a delay in initiating the urinary stream.

Decreased *force of urinary stream* or poor flow is the complaint of a slower stream than previously appreciated or a slower stream than their peers.

Intermittency is the complaint of urinary flow that stops and starts one or more times during the voiding phase.

Straining to void is the complaint of needing to exert effort by Valsalva, suprapubic pressure, or other means of increasing abdominal pressure in order to initiate or maintain the urinary stream.

Position-dependent micturition is the complaint of having to contort one's body into a specific position in order to improve the force of urinary stream or bladder emptying.

Incomplete bladder emptying is the complaint that the bladder is not empty immediately after voiding.

Double voiding or the need to immediately re-void is the complaint that further micturition is needed soon after voiding.

Post void dribbling is the complaint of involuntary urinary leakage immediately after voiding.

Urinary retention is the complaint of the persistent inability to pass urine.

Etiology of Obstructive Symptoms

The etiology of obstructive symptoms may be anatomic, secondary to an enlarged prostate gland in men, bladder neck obstruction, urethral stricture, urethral compression/fibrosis in women, or pelvic organ prolapse in women. The etiology of symptoms may also be functional, secondary to detrusor striated or smooth sphincter dyssynergia, a fixed bladder outlet, Fowler's syndrome in women, or poor bladder function (impaired bladder contractility). On occasion, LUTS suggestive of obstruction may exist in the absence of any anatomic or functional cause.

Increased outlet resistance is a much more common phenomenon in men than in women, with BPE being the leading cause. Benign prostatic hyperplasia (BPH)

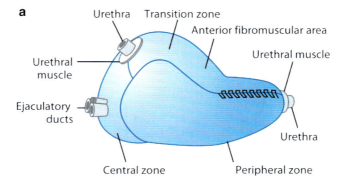

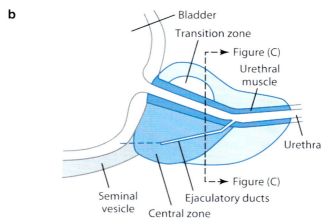

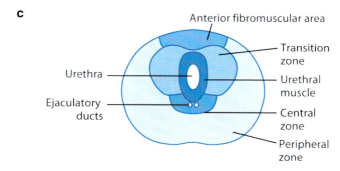

Fig. 10.1 Prostatic zonal anatomy (**a**) schematic, (**b**) sagittal cross-section, (**c**) transverse cross-section (adapted from Hanno et al. [5])

refers to typical histopathologic findings of glandular and stromal proliferation that occurs in nearly all men if they live long enough. The location of this growth within the prostate gland, surrounding and adjacent to the prostatic urethra (in the transitional and central zones), is what leads to voiding symptoms (Fig. 10.1). In many men however, the presence of BPH is confirmed pathologically in the absence of voiding symptoms. BPE refers to the increased size of the prostate but implies that a benign pathology has been confirmed. Benign prostatic obstruction (BPO) is a form of bladder outlet obstruction and this term is used when the cause of anatomic obstruction is known to be due to BPH. When histologic confirmation has not been made, preferred terminology is "LUTS suggestive of BPO" [7].

The prevalence of BPH on autopsy increases with age with 25% of men 40–50 years, 50% of men 50–60 years, 65% of men 60–70 years, 80% of men 70–80 years, and 90% of men 80–90 years showing histopathologic change [8]. Similarly, the prevalence of bothersome LUTS as measured by validated questionnaire, the American Urologic Association Symptom Score (AUASS), increases with advancing age [9]. However, clinical BPH varies widely with only a small percentage of those with histologic findings presenting for treatment of bothersome LUTS. Importantly, the size of the prostate gland is not linearly correlated to urodynamic evidence of obstruction or to severity of symptoms and therefore cannot be used as an indicator for treatment [10]. Similarly, small changes in prostatic size and tone can greatly improve LUTS thus explaining the large beneficial effects seen from medical management.

A basic evaluation of men presenting with LUTS should include a thorough medical history including the nature and duration of LUTS. Additional history should include any genital or sexual symptoms, prior urinary tract manipulation or surgery, and medication assessment. Physical exam should include a digital rectal exam to assess prostate size, consistency, presence of nodules, and anal sphincter tone. Palpation of the bladder to rule out distension should be performed and a basic neurologic assessment of motor and sensory function in the perineum and lower extremities is warranted. Urinalysis in the form of a dipstick should be carried out, with further evaluation if abnormalities are seen. In the evaluation of patients with LUTS suspected to be due to BPH there is no consensus on routine prostate-specific antigen (PSA) testing. Despite a lack of correlation between prostate symptoms, histology, size and even flow rate, an important relationship with PSA does exist. PSA, in men with BPH and no evidence of cancer, correlates with total prostate volume and is a predictor of the risk of acute urinary retention and ultimate need for surgery. Furthermore, it can be useful as a parameter for prognostic value for BPH progression and response to treatment [11–14]. Essentially, men with larger prostate glands and higher PSA values are at greater risk of experiencing further prostatic growth, worsening LUTS, progression to acute urinary retention and surgical intervention for their condition. Inevitably however, the routine use of PSA in this population will lead to several unnecessary prostate needle biopsies with their resultant complications, and diagnosis of clinically relevant and clinically irrelevant prostate cancer. The risks and benefits of PSA testing should be discussed with the patient.

A quantitative assessment of LUTS and degree of bother is recommended at the time of initial evaluation. The AUASS is a noninvasive, valid, reliable, and responsive index that correlates to the magnitude of urinary problems attributed to BPH (Table 10.2). A score of 7 points or less is considered mild LUTS, 8–19 points moderate LUTS, and 20–35 points severe LUTS. An addition quality of life measure

Table 10.2 American Urologic Association symptom index for benign prostatic hyperplasia (range from 0 to 35 points)

	Not at all	Less than 1 time in 5	Less than half the time	About half the time	More than half the time	Almost always
1. Over the last month how often have you had a sensation of not emptying your bladder completely after you finished urinating?	0	1	2	3	4	5
2. Over the last month how often have you had to urinate again less than 2 h after you finished urinating?	0	1	2	3	4	5
3. Over the last month how often have you found you stopped and started again several times while urinating?	0	1	2	3	4	5
4. Over the last month how often have you found it difficult to postpone urinating?	0	1	2	3	4	5
5. Over the last month how often have you had a weak stream while urinating?	0	1	2	3	4	5
6. Over the last month how often have you had to push or strain to begin urinating?	0	1	2	3	4	5
7. Over the last month how many times did you most typically get up to urinate from the time you went to bed until the time you got up in the morning?	0, none	1 time	2 times	3 times	4 times	5 or more times

AUA symptom index score: 0–7 mild, 8–18 moderate, 19–35 severe symptoms

	Quality of life due to urinary symptoms						Total
	Delighted	Pleased	Mostly satisfied	Mixed about equally satisfied and dissatisfied	Mostly dissatisfied	Unhappy	Terrible
1. If you were to spend the rest of your life with your urinary condition just the way it is now, how would you feel about that?	0	1	2	3	4	5	6

Quality of life assessment index (QOL) =

Quality of life assessment recommended by the World Health Organization

Adapted from Wein et al. [7]

allows for assessment of bother on a scale of 0–6 (delighted to terrible). This tool allows monitoring of symptoms over time, either in response to treatment or in the absence of treatment. The AUASS cannot be used as a diagnostic test or screening tool for BPH as it is nonspecific for BPH, in fact, women with OAB often attain very high scores. Neither PSA nor AUASS can replace a thorough history and physical exam in the evaluation of LUTS felt to be secondary to BPH.

A voiding diary should be completed by the patient to document the number of daily voids, the distribution of voids during the day and night, the volume voided, and fluid intake. Other parameters when present such as urgency and leakage of urine should also be documented.

The natural history of BPH is such that slow progression of symptoms over time is expected. Approximately 50% of the time patients with significant outlet obstruction develop overactive symptoms producing a combination of symptoms that exist during bladder filling and emptying. There has been a recent interest in initiating treatment to stabilize symptoms, reverse the natural progression of BPH, and avoid undesirable effects. Most men who seek treatment ultimately do so because of the bothersome nature of their symptoms which affects their quality of life. Treatment involves relief of the obstruction either by anatomic removal of the prostatic bulk or pharmacologic reduction in prostatic tone (alpha blockers) or size (5-alpha reductase inhibitors). Generally relief of obstruction results in diminution of OAB symptoms; although, these symptoms may return as the patient ages.

Primary bladder neck obstruction (PBNO) is a condition where the bladder neck fails to open adequately during voiding resulting in poor urinary flow [15, 16]. It is found most commonly in young to middle aged men, but may be seen in women and children as well [17, 18]. Symptoms are similar to those seen from prostatic obstruction, but on examination an enlarged prostate is not appreciated. In many situations patients go undiagnosed for many years and undergo multiple empiric treatments with various medications including antibiotics. The diagnosis is made urodynamically with confirmation of high pressure low flow voiding and fluoroscopic imaging confirming a failure of the bladder neck to relax with voiding (Fig. 10.2). Initial treatment includes a trial of alpha blockers; however, often definitive relief with transurethral incision of bladder neck (TUIBN) is needed.

Bladder neck contracture (BNC) is generally iatrogenic, occurring after radical prostatectomy, outlet reduction for BPO, transurethral resection of the prostate, or various other alternative strategies for treating BPO. The contracture is composed of scar tissue, preventing appropriate funneling of the bladder neck during voiding. The scar tissue may progress to complete luminal obliteration preventing any flow or urine or passage of instruments through the urethra. BNC rarely responds to medication therapy and commonly requires dilation or more definitive transurethral incision or resection of the bladder neck. Urethral stents have been used with mixed outcomes in attempts to avoid anastamotic urethroplasty, a technically challenging operation. The major risk of these interventions is urinary incontinence often requiring subsequent artificial urinary sphincter placement. This however should be delayed until confirmation of sustained opening of the contracture is confirmed. Recalcitrant contractures require major reconstructive surgery such as appendicovesicostomy,

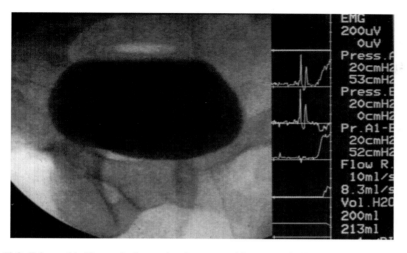

Fig. 10.2 Primary bladder neck obstruction documented fluoroscopically with failure of the bladder neck to funnel during voiding. A high pressure (52 cm H$_2$O) low flow (8.3 mL/s) pattern was seen on the urodynamic tracing

augmentation cystoplasty, and continent catheterizable stomas [19]. Chronic suprapubic tube drainage has been used as a less invasive means of management.

Urethral strictures can occur in men and women but are more common in men. They can result from urethral infections such as Chlamydia or gonorrhea or may result from prior urethral instrumentation or trauma [20]. Scar tissue narrows the urethral lumen and can vary in length from under a centimeter in length to several centimeters [21]. Progressive obstructive symptoms tend to develop with narrowing of the urinary stream, incomplete bladder emptying, and eventual acute urinary retention in some patients. Complications including urinary tract infection, prostatitis, epididymo-orchitis, bladder diverticuli, bladder stones, bladder wall thickening, and eventual bladder decompensation and hydroureteronephrosis can occur [22]. Left untreated, periurethral abscess formation with subsequent urethrocutaneous fistula formation to the perineum can occur. Urinary flow rate studies in patients with strictures generally show a low flow rate with a plateau pattern indicative of a slow protracted urine flow. Flow rates can also be helpful in detecting recurrent stricture in patients who have undergone previous successful treatment. Post void residual urine volumes are usually done concomitantly and together with flow rate provide a measure of voiding efficiency. Definitive diagnosis of a urethral stricture is made with either retrograde urethrogram (RUG) or cystoscopy. RUG combined with voiding images of the urethra can show the length as well as the caliber of the stricture. These studies are an important step in surgical planning for reconstruction of the urethra. Initial treatment generally involves dilation or incision of the stricture endoscopically with a direct visual internal urethrotomy (DVIU). But, less than half of patients will be cured with these interventions [21]. For patients who elect a more definitive primary therapy, urethroplasty can be a highly effective and cost effective option. Urethroplasty can be performed in an end to end fashion or augmented with buccal mucosa, penile skin or other flaps or grafts is generally recommended. Self catheterization or calibration can be an effective means of preventing recurrence and preventing future surgical intervention [23, 24]. However, patient compliance tends to limit the utility of this option. Urethral stents have won the favor of a few urologists with most others finding poor results, recurrent strictures, and great difficulty removing them should they wish to [25]. In patients who have failed multiple interventions including urethroplasty, perineal urethrostomy is a viable option that prevents the need for further surgery.

In women, bladder outlet obstruction may be the result of urethral compression from external vaginal cysts, urethral diverticuli, urethral strictures, or cancerous growths. It may also occur secondary to fibrosis of the urethra which prevents appropriate dilation and funneling during voiding and usually results from urethrovaginal atrophy. Pelvic organ prolapse can also produce anatomic obstruction due to kinking of the urethrovesical junction. Most commonly today, obstruction in the female is iatrogenic, secondary to treatment of urinary incontinence with various anti-incontinence procedures such as slings, retropubic suspensions, and urethral bulking agents. Vague symptoms may be present in women, often delaying diagnosis and confusing treatment. Urodynamics can be helpful, but no definitive pressure flow criteria exist to firmly diagnose obstruction in women. Alleviation of obstruction generally produces a marked improvement in voiding symptoms, but a high index of suspicion for obstruction must be present for proper diagnosis, especially in women who have undergone prior pelvic floor reconstruction. Urinary retention in young women in the absence of neurologic disease may be the result of *Fowler's syndrome*. Generally the condition comes on with symptoms of lower abdominal discomfort, inability to void for a day or more, and little urinary urgency or bladder sensation. Often these patients have concomitant polycystic ovarian syndrome. Patients are generally found to have over one liter of urine in their bladders and urodynamics show acontractility. A unique EMG abnormality is present that impairs sphincteric relaxation. The only successful treatment is neuromodulation; however, this is not effective in all patients [26].

Detrusor striated or smooth sphincter dyssynergia refer to phenomena in which the sphincteric mechanisms fail to normally relax(open) concomitant with bladder contraction, thereby preventing normal micturition and producing a functional obstruction to the flow of urine. Straited sphincter dyssynergia occurs almost exclusively in patients with suprasacral neurologic disease. During urodynamic studies an increase in pelvic floor EMG activity, rather than a decrease, in the presence of an obstructive voiding pattern is suggestive of this condition [27]. A non-neurogenic condition with similar findings termed Hinman's syndrome is felt to be the result of nonvoluntary contraction of the sphincteric mechanism during voiding. This is thought to be a learned behavior that can be unlearned with appropriate pelvic floor and biofeedback training. Smooth sphincter dysfunction, also referred to as bladder neck dysfunction, is seen almost exclusively in men and is generally not associated with neurologic disease, the notable exception being in both sexes with autonomic dysreflexia.

Fixed bladder outlet or resting residual sphincter tone is another neurologic phenomenon where the urethral smooth sphincter is competent, but non-relaxing and the striated sphincter is fixed thereby preventing funneling and opening of the urethra during voiding. Generally patients have mixed symptoms with incontinence and incomplete bladder emptying and their striated sphincter is not under voluntary control. Voiding generally occurs by Credé's maneuver [27]. A typical example is the myelodysplastic patient with neurogenic LUTS.

Bladder underactivity or poor bladder contractility may result from alternations in neuromuscular mechanisms necessary for initiating and maintaining a normal bladder (detrusor) contraction. Inhibition of the voiding reflex in a neurologically normal individual may also occur; it may be psychogenic or secondary to increased afferent input from the pelvic and perineal areas. Non-neurogenic causes also include impairment of bladder smooth muscle function which can result from over distension, drugs, severe infection, or fibrosis [28].

LUTS Suggestive of OAB

LUTS suggestive of OAB, previously referred to as irritative LUTS and now commonly referred to as OAB, occur during the filling/storage phase of micturition. Overactive symptoms increases with age in both men and women and consists of symptoms such as urgency, frequency of urination, nocturia, and urgency urinary incontinence (UUI).

OAB symptoms are described below [6].

Daytime urinary *frequency* is the complaint of more frequent micturition than previously considered normal.

Nocturia is the complaint of interruption of sleep one or more times due to the need to void.

Urgency is the complaint of a sudden, compelling desire to void which is difficult to defer.

Urgency urinary incontinence is the complaint of involuntary loss of urine associated with urgency.

Increased bladder sensation is the complaint of the desire to void at an earlier time point or smaller bladder volume than previously experienced.

Dysuria is the complaint of burning or discomfort during voiding.

Bladder pain is the compliant of suprapubic or retropubic pain, pressure, or discomfort, related to the bladder and usually increasing with bladder filling. It may persist or be relieved with bladder emptying. This is generally not a part of the OAB symptom complex.

Etiology of OAB Symptoms

OAB syndrome is the combination of urinary urgency, usually accompanied by frequency and nocturia, with or without UUI, in the absence of urinary tract infection or other obvious pathology [6]. Overactivity of the bladder during the filling/storage phase of micturition may be the result of involuntary bladder contractions, impaired detrusor compliance, or a combination of the two. Involuntary bladder contractions are commonly seen in the presence of neurologic disease, bladder outlet obstruction, SUI (presumably due to entry of urine into the proximal urethra eliciting a reflex bladder contraction), pelvic organ prolapse, bladder or ureteral calculi, urethral pathology, aging, increased afferent input secondary to inflammation or irritation, or may be truly idiopathic [28]. The involuntary muscle contraction may occur, in some individuals, as the result of release of excitatory neurotransmitters, specifically acetylcholine (Ach), from the urothelium during filling/storage [29]. Ach activates afferent nerve receptors leading to a premature or heightened sensation of distention or bladder fullness, urgency, or pain. In the setting of urgency incontinence it is generally believed that an involuntary contraction occurred precipitating the leakage. Urodynamics can confirm the presence of involuntary contractions, termed detrusor overactivity (DO); however, this imperfect test may show DO in the absence of clinically relevant symptoms and may fail to show DO when a very high index of suspicion exists. Furthermore, repeat studies are often inconsistent [30]. Several possible pathophysiologic mechanisms for OAB have been described including (1) reduced suprapontine inhibition, (2) damaged axonal paths in the spinal cord, (3) damaged peripheral neuronal paths, (4) loss of peripheral inhibition, (5) enhancement of excitatory neurotransmission in the micturition reflex pathway, (6) increased afferent input, and (7) idiopathic [2]. Decreased compliance is usually the sequelae of neurologic disease but may also result from any process that destroys the elastic or viscoelastic properties of the bladder wall.

A basic evaluation of patients presenting with overactive LUTS should include a thorough medical history including the nature and duration of symptoms. Additional history should include any genital or sexual symptoms, prior urinary tract manipulation or surgery, gross hematuria, smoking history, and medication assessment. Physical exam should include a digital rectal exam in men to assess prostate size, consistency, presence of nodules, and anal sphincter tone and a pelvic examination in women to assess degree of uterine or bladder prolapse, urethral hypermobility, and pelvic mass. Palpation of the bladder to rule out distension should be performed and a basic neurologic assessment of motor and sensory function of the perineum and lower extremities is warranted. Urinalysis in the form of a dipstick should be instituted with further evaluation if abnormalities are seen. Persistent overactive symptoms should be evaluated with urine cytology with consideration of cystoscopy.

A voiding diary should be completed by the patient to document the number of daily voids, the distribution of voids during the day and night, the volume voided, and fluid intake. Other parameters when present such as urgency and leakage of urine should also be documented. Several validated questionnaires exist and are generally helpful to evaluate initial symptom severity and bother and the patient's response to treatment.

Treatment for these conditions is aimed at decreasing bladder activity or increasing bladder capacity generally through behavioral modifications such as timed voiding, Kegel exercises, fluid restriction, and avoidance of bladder irritants. Medication therapy with antimuscarinic drugs is added when the patient has significant bother or symptoms refractory to conservative measures.

A less common cause of urinary frequency or nocturia is *polyuria*. Polyuria refers to an increase in the volume of urine excreted on a daily basis. The etiologic mechanisms include increased fluid intake (polydipsia, psychogenic polydipsia), exogenous or endogenous diuretics, and abnormal states of central or peripheral osmoregulation. Nocturnal polyuria refers to a disproportionate amount of urine excreted overnight compared to during the day. A decrease in nighttime antidiuretic hormone secretion is a common culprit among the elderly [31].

Increased bladder sensation or bladder pain may be the result of bladder pain syndrome/interstitial cystitis (BPS/IC). This clinical diagnosis is made after ruling out other causes of lower urinary tract discomfort. BPS/IC is defined as "an unpleasant sensation (pain, pressure, discomfort) perceived to be related to the urinary bladder, associated with lower urinary tract symptoms of more than 6 weeks duration, in the absence of infection or other identifiable cause" [32]. Therapy is aimed at increasing bladder capacity or decreasing sensory (afferent) input.

Incontinence

Urinary incontinence is defined as the involuntary loss of urine and generally occurs during the filling/storage phase of micturition. Incontinence symptoms increase with age in both men and women and consist of complaints such as stress related urinary incontinence, urgency urinary incontinence, and insensible urine loss.

Incontinent urinary symptoms are described below [6].

Urinary incontinence is the complaint of involuntary loss of urine.

Stress incontinence is the complaint of involuntary loss of urine during coughing, sneezing, or physical exertion.

Urgency incontinence is the complaint of involuntary loss of urine associated with urgency.

Mixed urinary incontinence is the complaint of involuntary loss of urine during coughing, sneezing, or physical exertion (SUI) and with urgency (UUI).

Postural incontinence is the complaint of involuntary loss of urine associated with change in body position.

Nocturnal enuresis is the complaint of involuntary loss of urine during sleep.

Continuous incontinence is the compliant of continuous involuntary loss of urine.

Insensible incontinence is the complaint of urine loss without awareness.

Coital incontinence is the complaint of involuntary loss of urine with intercourse.

Table 10.3 Classification of the etiologies of incontinence

I. Urethral incontinence
   A. Bladder dysfunction/detrusor overactivity
      1. Involuntary contractions
      2. Impaired compliance
   B. Urethral dysfunction/outlet underactivity
      1. Urethral hypermobility
      2. Intrinsic sphincter deficiency
   C. Functional
      1. Secondary to functional disability
      2. Secondary to cognitive impairment
II. Extraurethral incontinence
   A. Fistula
      1. Vesicovaginal
      2. Ureterovaginal
      3. Urethrovaginal
      4. Rectourethral
   B. Ectopic ureter

Etiology of Incontinence

The etiology of incontinence varies by type. The two main categories are bladder dysfunction or detrusor overactivity and urethral dysfunction or outlet underactivity. A simple classification scheme is shown in Table 10.3. Detrusor overactivity may be due to neurologic disease or may exist with or may be due to bladder outlet obstruction, inflammation, or be idiopathic. The result may be involuntary bladder contractions that produce associated leakage of urine or impaired compliance producing an elevation in detrusor pressure that exceeds urethral pressure leading to incontinence. Decreased outlet resistance may result from any process that damages the innervations or structural elements of the smooth and/or striated sphincter (intrinsic sphincter deficiency (ISD)) or support of the bladder outlet in the female (urethral hypermobility). This may occur with neurologic disease, surgical or mechanical (obstetric) trauma, or aging [28]. Additionally, incontinence may be the result of functional or cognitive impairment or abnormal urinary tract communication.

SUI in the female was classically divided into two relatively discreet entities: urethral hypermobility and ISD. Hypermobility of the bladder outlet was felt to be due to poor bladder support such that during episodes of increase intra-abdominal pressure, mobility of the outlet led to loss of competence and urinary leakage. ISD is the loss of urethral competence, specifically the sphincter mechanism, such that closure pressure cannot overcome bladder pressure in certain situations [28].

These categories are considered less discrete today with the contemporary view favoring that varying degrees of each component are present in most women with SUI. Furthermore, the need for this type of discreet classification has lost its value as treatments are no longer exclusive to one entity or the other. In general, today, treatment is the same for both underlying etiologies. In theory, outlet related incontinence in the male should be similar to the female; however, hypermobility of the bladder neck and urethra has not been found as an etiology in the male. ISD in the male is felt to be the result of neurologic disease, surgical or mechanical trauma, or aging, with treatment of prostatic diseases the most common underlying cause.

UUI is described in the section on overactive LUTS above.

MUI generally results from combined deficits leading to both SUI and UUI. Combination therapy addressing each component is generally most efficacious.

Nocturnal enuresis in isolation is most commonly seen in children. In adults it may be a component of the OAB syndrome and essentially due to UUI while sleeping. It can also be the result of oversedation caused by sleep aids and other psychotropic drugs. In the setting of nocturnal polyuria, nocturnal enuresis may occur due to excessive nighttime urine output. Conservative measures such as nighttime alarms to wake the patient prior to a leakage episode, fluid restriction, and treatment of lower extremity edema if present, are generally first line. When these therapies fail antidiuretic hormone may be prescribed in order to decrease nighttime urine production.

Continuous incontinence can be the result of a urinary tract fistula, urethral erosion, overflow incontinence. Treatment of the urinary tract fistula will often cure the patient of their incontinence; however, a high index of suspicion to make the diagnosis is necessary. Urethral erosion generally occurs in the setting of a long term indwelling catheter. Commonly, the patients affected have a neurologic condition that lead to urinary retention precipitating the initial placement of the catheter. Urethral reconstruction can be attempted in these patients, but generally bladder neck closure with diversion of urine is needed. Overflow incontinence is generally the result of bladder outlet obstruction and relief of the incontinence relies on effective management of the primary problem. For some patients self intermittent catheterization can ameliorate symptoms and provide a relatively noninvasive treatment option.

Insensible incontinence may occur in the neurogenic population, the elderly, or the very young. Patient report no sensation of urine loss but have the feeling of wetness. This type of incontinence can be the most challenging as it often does not respond to any of the aforementioned treatment strategies. When all else fails options such as bladder neck closure with suprapubic tube placement, ileal chimney, and continent catheterizable reservoir's can be discussed with the patient.

Coital incontinence may occur due to SUI or UUI during intercourse or at the time of orgasm. Though the topic is controversial and little high quality data exists, a recent editorial summarizing the available evidence suggests that, "[coital incontinence] could be two separate entities: if leakage occurs at penetration, it can be almost invariably the consequence of an anatomic defect, while coital incontinence at orgasm may more frequently be related to an involuntary detrusor contraction either triggered by orgasm or by urethral instability due to sphincteric deficiency" [33]. It is uncommon for this coital incontinence to exist in isolation and generally treatment is based on concomitant symptoms and severity.

References

1. Wein AJ, Levin RM, Barrett DM. Voiding function: relevant anatomy, physiology, and pharmacology. In: Duckett JW, Howards ST, Grayhack JT, Gillenwater JY, editors. Adult and pediatric urology. St. Louis: Mosby; 1991. p. 933–99.
2. Wein AJ. Pathophysiology and classification of lower urinary tract dysfunction: overview. In: Wein AJ, Kavoussi LR, Novick AC, Partin AW, Peters CA, editors. Campbell-Walsh urology. 10th ed. Philadelphia: Elsevier Saunders; 2011. p. 1834–46.
3. Abrams P. New words for old: lower urinary tract symptoms for "prostatism". BMJ. 1994;308(6934):929–30.
4. Stewart WF, Van Rooyen JB, Cundiff GW, Abrams P, Herzog AR, Corey R, Hunt TL, Wein AJ. Prevalence and burden of overactive bladder in the United States. World J Urol. 2003;20(6):327–36.
5. Irwin DE, Milsom I, Hunskaar S, et al. Population-based survey of urinary incontinence, overactive bladder, and other lower urinary tract symptoms in five countries: results of the EPIC study. Eur Urol. 2006;50(6):1306–14; discussion 1314–5.
6. Haylen BT, de Ridder D, Freeman RM, Swift SE, Berghmans B, Lee J, Monga A, Petri E, Rizk DE, Sand PK, Schaer GN. International Urogynecological Association, International Continence Society. An International Urogynecological Association (IUGA)/International Continence Society (ICS) joint report on the terminology for female pelvic floor dysfunction. Neurourol Urodyn. 2010;29(1):4–20.
7. Wein AJ, Lee DI. Benign prostatic hyperplasia and related entities. In: Hanno PH, Malkokwicz SB, Wein AJ, editors. Penn clinical manual of urology. Philadelphia: Elsevier; 2007. p. 479–521.
8. Guess HA, Arrighi HM, Metter EJ, Fozard JL. Cumulative prevalence of prostatism matches the autopsy prevalence of benign prostatic hyperplasia. Prostate. 1990;17(3):241–6.
9. Oishi K, Boyle P, Barry M, et al. Epidemiology and natural history of benign prostatic hyperplasia. In: 4th International Consultation on Benign Prostatic Hyperplasia. Plymouth (UK): Plymbridge Distributors Ltd; 1998.p. 23–59.
10. Blaivas JG. The bladder is an unreliable witness. Neurourol Urodyn. 1996;15(5):443–5.
11. Cg R. The utility of serum prostatic-specific antigen in the management of men with benign prostatic hyperplasia. Int J Impot Res. 2008;20 Suppl 3:S19–26.
12. Bohnen AM, Groeneveld FP, Bosch JL. Serum prostate-specific antigen as a predictor of prostate volume in the community: the Krimpen study. Eur Urol. 2007;51(6):1645–52; discussion 1652–3.
13. Cg R. BPH progression: concept and key learning from MTOPS, ALTESS, COMBAT, and ALF-ONE. BJU Int. 2008;101 Suppl 3:17–21.
14. Lieber MM, Roberts RO. Prostate volume and prostate specific antigen in the absence of prostate cancer: a review of the relationship and prediction of long-term outcomes. Prostate. 2001;49(3):208–12.
15. Marion G. Surgery of the neck of the bladder. B J Urol. 1933;5:351–7.
16. Turner-Warwick R, Whiteside CG, Worth PHL, et al. A urodynamic view of the clinical problems associated with bladder neck dysfunction and its treatment by endoscopic incision and transtrigonal posterior prostatectomy. B J Urol. 1973;45:44–59.
17. Diokno AC. HJ, Bennett CJ. Bladder neck obstruction in women: a real entity. J Urol. 1984;132:294–8.
18. Smey P, King LR, Firlit CF. Dysfunctional voiding in children secondary to internal sphincter dyssynergia: treatment with phenoxybenzamine. Urol Clin North Am. 1980;7:337–47.
19. Westney OL. Salvage surgery for bladder outlet obstruction after prostatectomy or cystectomy. Curr Opin Urol. 2008;18(6):570–4.
20. Beard DE, Goodyear WE. Urethral stricture: a pathological study. J Urol. 1948;59:619–26.
21. Mundy AR, Andrich DE. Urethral strictures. BJU Int. 2011;107(1):6–26.

22. Romero Perez P, Mira Llinaries A. Complications of the lower urinary tract secondary to urethral stenosis. Actas Urol Esp. 1996;20:786–93.
23. Harriss DR, Beckingham IJ, Lemberger RJ, Lawrence WT. Long-term results of intermittent low-friction selfcathetersation in patients with recurrent urethral strictures. Br J Urol. 1994;74:790–2.
24. Smith AL, Ferlise VJ, Rovner ES. Female urethral strictures: successful management with long-term clean intermittent catheterization after urethral dilatation. BJU Int. 2006;98(1):96–9.
25. Palminteri E. Stents and urethral strictures: a lesson learned? Eur Urol. 2008;54:498–500.
26. Kavia RB, Datta SN, Dasgupta R, Elneil S, Fowler CJ. Urinary retention in women: its causes and management. BJU Int. 2006;97(2):281–7.
27. Wein AJ. Lower urinary tract dysfunction in neurologic injury and disease. In: Wein AJ, Kavoussi LR, Novick AC, Partin AW, Peters CA, editors. Campbell-Walsh urology. Philadelphia: Saunders; 2007. p. 2011–44.
28. Wein AJ, Moy ML. Voiding function and dysfunction; urinary incontinence. In: Hanno PH, Malkokwicz SB, Wein AJ, editors. Penn clinical manual of urology. Philadelphia: Elsevier; 2007. p. 341–478.
29. Andersson K-E, Chapple CR, Cardozo L, et al. Pharmacological treatment of urinary incontinence. In: Abrams P, Cardozo L, Khoury S et al., editors. Incontinence. 4th ed. Paris: Health Publications Ltd; 2009. p. 631–99.
30. Abrams P, Drake M. Overactive bladder. In: Wein AJ, Kavoussi LR, Novick AC, Partin AW, Peters CA, editors. Campbell-Walsh urology. Philadelphia: Saunders; 2007. p. 2079–90.
31. Hirayama A, Torimoto K, Yamada A, Tanaka N, Fujimoto K, Yoshida K, Hirao Y. Relationship between nocturnal urine volume, leg edema, and urinary antidiuretic hormone in older men. Urology. 2011;77(6):1426–31.
32. Hanno PM, Burks DA, Clemens JQ, Dmochowski RR, Erickson D, Fitzgerald MP, et al. AUA guideline for the diagnosis and treatment of interstitial cystitis/bladder pain syndrome. J Urol. 2011;185(6):2162–70.
33. Serati M, Cattoni E, Braga A, Siesto G, Salvatore S. Coital incontinence: relation to detrusor overactivity and stress incontinence. A controversial topic. Neurourol Urodyn. 2011;30(8):1415.

Chapter 11
Geriatric Sexuality

Philip T. Zhao, Daniel Su, and Allen D. Seftel

Introduction

The older population of the United States, focusing upon persons aged 65 years or beyond numbered 39.6 million in 2009 and is expected to rise significantly to almost 55 million by 2020 [1]. Knowledge regarding sexuality amongst older Americans is limited as it encompasses aspects including function, behavioral activity, partnership attitudes, and general health [2]. As men and women grow older, they are more susceptible to medical pathologies that can affect sexual health. Although illness and increasing age can decrease the prevalence of sexual activity, numerous studies show that a substantial number of older people engage in intercourse and sexual behavior even into their eighth and ninth decade of life. In a landmark study, Laumann et al. [3] detailed both male and female sexual dysfunction (FSD) in a younger cohort of men and women. Analysis of data came from the National Health and Social Life Survey, a probability sample study of sexual behavior in a demographically representative, 1992 cohort of the US adults. A national probability sample of 1,749 women and 1,410 men aged 18–59 years at the time of the survey, participated. Sexual dysfunction was more prevalent for women (43%) than men (31%) and was associated with various demographic characteristics, including age and educational attainment. Lindau et al., examining an older cohort, reported that the frequency of sexual

---

Fifty marks the beginning of the best years of our lives, including the best sex of our lives (Dr. Christiane Northrup)

P.T. Zhao • D. Su
Department of Surgery, Division of Urology, UMDNJ-Robert Wood Johnson
Medical School, New Brunswick, NJ 08901, USA

A.D. Seftel (✉)
Department of Surgery, Division of Urology, Cooper Medical School of Rowan University,
Camden, NJ 08103, USA
e-mail: seftel-allen@cooperhealth.edu

T.J. Guzzo et al. (eds.), *Primer of Geriatric Urology*, DOI 10.1007/978-1-4614-4773-3_11,   143
© Springer Science+Business Media New York 2013

activity in people up to 74 years of age was similar to that reported amongst adults 18–59 in the 1992 National Health and Social Life Survey, despite a significantly higher ratio (>50%) of bothersome sexual problems [4].

As a result of significant bothersome sexual problems and misconceptions about aging and sex, a quarter of sexually active older adults refrain from sexual activity and many of them do not discuss these issues with their physicians. Although there exists a massive and growing market for drugs and devices to improve sexual function and decrease morbidities amongst the geriatric population, medication and surgery may not be suited for everyone. Therefore, physician knowledge and patient education should play an active role in improving patient counseling and addressing potentially treatable sexual problems.

Sexual Myths of Aging

A significant part of the barrier to adequately diagnosing and treating sexual conditions in older adults is the perpetual myths regarding sex in aging individuals—that the stereotypical old person is slow moving, slow thinking, and rarely explores or indulges in his or her sexuality. Contrary to widely held beliefs and cultural and social views, the aging population continues to enjoy their sexuality. Common myths include the fact that erectile dysfunction (ED) is a normal part of aging, that old people do not have sexual desires or capabilities, and that the elderly are too frail to attempt intercourse or perverse when they do have no basis in reality [5]. In addition, the media has perpetuated some of these stereotypes of "dirty old men" and portrayed the elderly in a negative light when it comes to their sexuality [5]. They do a disservice not only to the large portion of the country's population who are elderly but also to the medical professionals who help and treat older patients. In order to build a healthy society and integrate our increasingly older population, the public should be open-minded and tolerant of its aging citizens in regards to their sexuality.

There are factors intertwined with aging that effect sexuality that cross gender lines. Many of these issues impact both men and women during the aging process. There are life stressors such as career, finance, physical and mental fatigue, and drug and alcohol abuse that can affect sexuality tremendously [6].

There exist significant emotional and life cycle disparities between men and women as they grow older. Older men generally are more prone to be involved in a relationship than their female counterparts; a study shows that 78% of men aged 75–85 were in a spousal or sexual relationship compared to 40% of the women in the same age group [4]. This wide gap can be attributed to several factors including the age structure. Women were also more likely to rate sex as an unimportant part of life and relationships versus men. A multinational survey of people aged 40–80 years of age shows that women prioritize cognitive and emotional aspects of sexuality as well as general happiness as a more important component of subjective sexual wellbeing [7]. Women also reported a higher proportion of lack of pleasure with sex. Despite the fact that bothersome sexual problems affect men and women equally, women were less likely than men to discuss these problems with their physicians [8]. Issues include patient unwillingness to initiate discussion, poor general communication with the doctor, sex and age differences between the patient and physician, and negative social attitudes about women's sexuality especially at older age [9, 10].

The Sexual Response Cycle in the Aging Patient

The four stages of sexual response cycle change as people grow older—excitement, plateau, orgasm, and resolution [11, 12]. Excitement depends on a multitude of visual, olfactory, auditory, and memory stimuli. Plateau is defined as the maintenance and intensification of arousal. Orgasm involves the rhythmic muscular contractions typical of climax. Resolution is the state of relaxation after orgasm.

These stages change dramatically as men and women age and they impact sexuality at every level [13]. For women, there is elongation of the excitement and plateau stages as they age. This is associated with increased time to attain sufficient vaginal lubrication, as there is a marked decrease in production of lubrication. Orgasmic contractions decrease in quantity and intensity, as there is atrophy of the vaginal mucosa and reduced elasticity and muscle tone. There is also a sharp decrease in the length of the resolution stage. Anatomically, there is significant atrophy of the vaginal tissues, decreased vaginal canal length and width, loss of vulvar tissue, and decrease in size of the clitoris. Estrogen levels fall sharply and play a dominant role in changes in female sexual function after menopause. In some women after menopause, the loss of reproductive capacity either diminishes interest in sexual intercourse or increases the eagerness to engage in sexual activities because the fear of pregnancy is gone [13].

In the elderly male [14], all four stages of sexual response decrease as men age. More time is required for penile stimulation in order to obtain and maintain a sufficient erection to engage in sex. There is a prolongation of the plateau phase with a shorter transition from orgasm to ejaculation. Orgasms become weaker with shorter intervals and smaller contractions. There is also a significant reduction in the amount of semen volume compared with younger men [15]. Penile detumescence occurs more frequently and rapidly in the resolution phase and there is a prolonged refractory period between erections [16]. Of course, all of these changes occur in conjunction with decreasing levels of testosterone, which is a primary driver of sexual desire and perhaps function in males.

Psychological Issues

Psychological issues that impact sexuality in the aging population are lifetime sexual experiences, levels of satisfaction pertaining to life, self-esteem and confidence levels, body images, and general attitudes towards sex. Historically, living arrangements and loss of a spouse or significant other have presented challenges and psychologic issues to the surviving partner regarding future sexual relationships [17]. Depression affects both males and females and can have lasting psychologic implications that substantially decrease interest and ability to engage in a sexual relationship [17].

The Epidemiology of Sexual Dysfunction in the Aging Patient

The description of the incidence and prevalence of sexuality of the aging population is relatively recent. This barrier to accumulating these data include the sensitivity of the subject matter, the difficulties in conducting what may potentially be embarrassing interviews, the poor response rate from surveys and self-reporting biases. In addition to the Laumann and Lindau studies discussed above, a large, well-done recent report is The Global Study of Sexual Attitudes and Behaviors [7]. This large, multinational study collected data from 27,500 men and women aged 40–80 years of age using standardized questionnaires. The authors found that more than 80% of men and 65% of women had sexual intercourse during the past year. The most common sexual dysfunctions for men were early ejaculation (14%) and erectile dysfunction (10%). For women, the lack of sexual desire (21%), inability to reach orgasm (16%), and inadequate lubrication (16%) were most common sexual problems. Overall 28% of men and 39% of women were affected by at least one sexual dysfunction. This study found that sexual desire and activity are in fact widespread amongst the elderly population; the prevalence of sexual dysfunction was quite high and tends to increase with age, especially in men.

Sexual Dysfunction in the Aging Female

The incidence of sexual dysfunction in the aging female has been much harder to characterize. This is mostly due to the ambiguity in the diagnosis of FSD. Laumann et al. [3] analyzed data from the National Health and Social Life Survey, a probability sample study of sexual behavior in a demographically representative, 1992 cohort of the US adults. A national probability sample of 1,749 women and 1,410 men aged 18–59 years at the time of the survey, demonstrated that 43% of women surveyed had sexual dysfunction. With respect to women in this study, the data demonstrated an unaffected group (58% prevalence), a low sexual desire category (22% prevalence), a category for arousal problems (14% prevalence), and a group with sexual pain (7% prevalence).

The Global Study of Sexual Attitudes and Behaviors [7] multinational study collected data from 27,500 men and women aged 40–80 years of age using standardized questionnaires. The study results found that for women, the lack of sexual desire (21%), the inability to reach orgasm (16%), and inadequate lubrication (16%) were the most common sexual problems. There are limited quantitative or qualitative criteria for diagnosis of FSD. There are data however supporting vaginal atrophy as a cause for not only sexual dysfunction but also voiding dysfunction, along with issues with emotional wellbeing and routine activity in the postmenopausal female [18].

A recent study sought to estimate the prevalence of low sexual desire and hypoactive sexual desire disorder (HSDD) in the US women, focusing on their menopausal status [19]. The authors performed a cross-sectional study. From a probability sample of households, 2,207 US women aged 30–70 years and in stable relationships (>or=3 months) were interviewed by telephone. The analysis focused on 755 premenopausal women and 552 naturally and 637 surgically menopausal women. Low sexual desire was defined using the Profile of Female Sexual Function desire domain, and HSDD was defined using the Profile of Female Sexual Function and the Personal Distress Scale. The prevalence of low sexual desire ranged from 26.7% among premenopausal women to 52.4% among naturally menopausal women. The prevalence of HSDD was highest among surgically menopausal women (12.5%). Compared with premenopausal women and adjusting for age, race/ethnicity, educational level, and smoking status, the prevalence ratios for HSDD were 2.3 (95% confidence interval, 1.2–4.5) for surgically menopausal women and 1.2 (0.5–2.8) for naturally menopausal women; the prevalence ratios for low sexual desire were 1.3 (0.9–1.9) and 1.5 (1.0–2.2) for surgically and naturally menopausal women, respectively.

Recent data from the Rancho Bernardo study were supportive of these findings. A total of 1,303 older women from the Rancho Bernardo Study were mailed a questionnaire on general health, recent sexual activity, sexual satisfaction, along with the Female Sexual Function Index (FSFI) questionnaire. A total of 806 of 921 respondents (87.5%) aged 40 years or more answered questions about recent sexual activity. Their median age was 67 years; mean years since menopause was 25; most were upper middle class; 57% had attended at least 1 year of college; and 90% reported good to excellent health. Half (49.8%) reported sexual activity within the past month with or without a partner, the majority of whom reported arousal (64.5%), lubrication (69%), and orgasm (67.1%) at least most of the time, although one third reported low, very low, or no sexual desire. Although frequency of arousal, lubrication, and orgasm decreased with age, the youngest (<55 years) and oldest (>80 years) women reported a higher frequency of orgasm satisfaction. Emotional closeness during sex was associated with more frequent arousal, lubrication, and orgasm; estrogen therapy was not. Overall, two thirds of sexually active women were moderately or very satisfied with their sex life, as were almost half of sexually inactive women [20].

Hormonal issues in the female: Menopause

Menopause is defined as the permanent cessation of menses occurring usually between the ages of 45 and 55 with estrogen deficiency as the primary diagnostic criterion [18, 21]. Its symptoms include hot flashes, sexual dysfunction, mood disorders, and urogenital symptoms and it increases the risk for cardiovascular, musculoskeletal, and psychogenic sequelae. Diagnosis is usually made in women with follicle-stimulating hormone (FSH) levels greater than 40, although FSH is not the most accurate way to assess menopausal status as FSH levels may vary considerably from the transition to pre- and perimenopause to menopause [18]. If menopause occurs before the age of 40, it is considered pathologic and a workup should be initiated. This is considered premature ovarian failure and is usually secondary to autoimmune oophoritis [18]. Bilateral oophorectomy can also induce menopause.

Although the changes brought on by menopause are, for the most part, considered adverse, some women feel relaxed and liberated from the fear of pregnancy. Others experience a psychologic decrease of what they consider as their sexuality and femininity. The vaginal changes associated with menopause can cause dyspareunia and worsen the sexual experience. Lower estrogen levels also predispose menopausal women to atrophic vaginitis and more frequent vaginal infections which are associated with itching, burning, and discharge [18, 21].

Although estrogen replacement therapy (ERT) had been the mainstay of treatment for menopausal women for decades under the premise that it safeguards against osteoporosis and cardiovascular disease, new data (The Women's Health Initiative E-Alone Trial) revealed that ERT may result in increased cardiac events and cerebrovascular disease in healthy women as well as an increased risk of venous thromboembolism [22]. There was also concern regarding ERT predisposing women to higher risks for breast and uterine cancers [23]. Thus, the current focus is on treating the sequelae of symptoms such as osteoporosis, postmenopausal depression, and sexual dysfunctions, without the use of ERT.

Sexual Dysfunction in the Aging Male: Erectile Dysfunction, Ejaculatory Dysfunction, and Hormonal Issues in the Male

Epidemiology: Erectile dysfunction, the inability to achieve or maintain an erection sufficient for sexual activity has been thought to account for the majority of sexual dysfunction in the aging male. Approximately 152 million men worldwide and as many as 30 million American men are affected by erectile dysfunction. As many as 322 million men worldwide are projected to have erectile dysfunction by 2,025 [24, 25]. It is estimated that prevalence of erectile dysfunction is approximately 20% in men age 50–59 years of age. Eighteen million American men 40–70 years of age are estimated to be affected with some degree of erectile dysfunction [24, 25]. It has also been demonstrated that prevalence of erectile dysfunction increases with age [25–28]. Based on the Massachusetts Male Aging Study [28], one of several large, well done, epidemiologic studies on this topic, the crude incidence rate of erectile dysfunction was 25.9 cases per 1,000 man-years. The annual incidence rate increases with each decade of age and was 12.4 cases per 1,000 man-years for American men 40–49 years of age, 29.8 for men 50–59 years of age, and 46.5 for men 60–69 years of age ([28], Fig 11.1).

Ejaculatory dysfunction: Ejaculatory dysfunction in the aging male can be manifest as either rapid or delayed ejaculation. Both entities are difficult to quantitate epidemiologically. Delayed ejaculation, (which is not well-defined in terms of time),

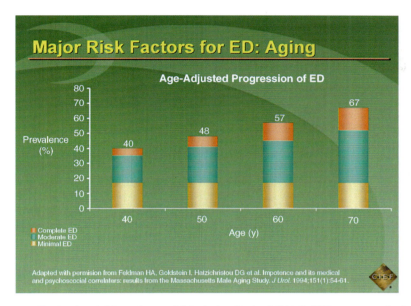

Fig. 11.1 The landmark Massachusetts Male Aging Study (MMAS) [28], a community-based observational study of nearly 3,000 men, aged 40–70 years, clearly established that ED is highly prevalent, age-related, and progressive. Subjects ($n = 1,290$) were asked to respond to a sexual activity questionnaire characterizing their level of ED. *Minimal* ED was defined as "usually able to get or keep an erection"; *moderate*, as "sometimes able"; and *complete*, as "never able to get and keep an erection" [1]. Self-rated ED was reflected by higher frequency of erectile difficulty during intercourse, lower monthly rates of sexual activity and erection, and lower satisfaction with sex life and partner. In the MMAS study, 40% of men were estimated to have ED at age 40, but this increased to 67% at age 70. Age was the only variable that proved to be a statistically significant predictor of ED ($P < 0.0001$) (courtesy of testosteroneupdate.org.)

in the aging male is most likely a combination of neuropathy of the ejaculatory pathway and a change in the prostatic milieu. The neuropathy may result from diabetes, vitamin deficiency, anatomic spine issues, CNS issues, thyroid issues, post-transurethral resection of the prostate, any pelvic surgery that affects the pelvic nerves such as radical prostatectomy, or combinations thereof. The prostate is predominately a reproductive organ in the young man, and turns into a less glandular, more fibrotic organ with aging, and thus is less secretory. This may result in "delayed" ejaculation, wherein ejaculation is delayed. In the young man, nonorganic, delayed ejaculation is also thought to be psychogenic in origin, while it is assumed that this is less likely in the older man. In general, delayed ejaculation is challenging to treat, as many of the disease processes noted above are chronic, rendering correction of the delayed ejaculation less likely.

Premature ejaculation in the aging male is also enigmatic [29]. The definition of premature ejaculation is somewhat elusive as worldwide studies reflect the disparity in the "normal" ejaculatory period [30]. In a large, multinational study, the intravaginal latency time (the IELT, which is the sine qua nonmeasurement for rapid ejaculation), had a positively skewed distribution, with a geometric mean of 5.7 min and a median of 6.0 min (range: 0.1–52.1 min). Men from Turkey had the shortest median IELT (4.4 min). Men from the United Kingdom had the longest IELT (10.0 min). Circumcision and condom use had no significant impact on the median IELT. Subjects who were discontent with their latency time had slightly lower median IELT values of 5.2 min than the median of the population.

Premature or rapid ejaculation has been historically defined by time. Ejaculation within 1–2 min of erection, combined with distress, is felt to be the two components of the current definition. This definition of rapid ejaculation can be independent of vaginal penetration, in spite of the fact that intravaginal latency time is used as the barometer of rapid ejaculation [31].

Please recall the following data discussed earlier. Laumann et al. [3] detailed both male and FSD in a younger cohort of men and women. Analysis of data came from the National Health and Social Life Survey, a probability sample study of sexual behavior in a demographically representative, 1992 cohort of the US adults. A national probability sample of 1,749 women and 1,410 men aged 18–59 years at the time of the survey, participated. Sexual dysfunction was more prevalent for women (43%) than men (31%) and was associated with various demographic characteristics, including age and educational attainment. The most common sexual dysfunction in this youngish male cohort was premature ejaculation.

Rapid ejaculation may be a response to erectile dysfunction and may therefore correct itself once the ED is corrected. Alternatively, rapid ejaculation may be lifelong and may only rise to the surface as a problem for the aging male. Rapid ejaculation is thought to be in part genetic in the young man. Jern et al. noted a moderate genetic influence (28%) in rapid ejaculation in a population-based sample of 1,196 Finnish male twins, age 33–43 years. [32]. This genetic relationship has not been established in the aging male.

Hormonal issues: Hormonal issues in the aging male affect sexual desire, erections, and ejaculation [33]. The most common male hormonal issues are related to low testosterone. Other disorders are less common such as thyroid disorders. While data are limited regarding thyroid disorders, however a recent study offered the following data: 48 adult men, 34 with hyperthyroidism, and 14 with hypothyroidism were studied. The mean age of the enrolled subjects was 43.2 +/−12.1 years (range, 22–62 years). No significant difference was found in the age at presentation between hyperthyroid ($n = 34$) and hypothyroid ($n = 14$) patients. In hyperthyroid men, the prevalence of hypoactive sexual desire, delayed ejaculation, premature ejaculation, and ED was 17.6, 2.9, 50, and 14.7%, whereas in hypothyroid men, the prevalence of HSD, DE, and ED was 64.3% and of PE was 7.1%. After thyroid hormone normalization in hyperthyroid subjects, PE prevalence fell from 50 to 15%, whereas DE was improved in half of the treated hypothyroid men. Ejaculation latency time doubled after treatment of hyperthyroidism (from 2.4 +/− 2.1 to 4.0 +/− 2.0 min), whereas for hypothyroid men it declined significantly, from 21.8 +/− 10.9 to 7.4 +/− 7.2 ($P < 0.01$ for both). The cohort in this study was a bit younger, mean age 43, and thus the results may not be fully translatable to the older male [34].

Serum testosterone declines with aging in the male. This decline, termed Testosterone Deficiency (TD) or hypogonadism, in the aging male, is the subject of major interest. Testosterone deficiency in aging men is a condition associated with decreased sexual satisfaction and a decline of general wellbeing. The definition of hypogonadism is as follows [35]: Hypogonadism in men is a clinical syndrome that results from failure of the testis to produce physiological levels of testosterone (androgen deficiency) and a normal number of spermatozoa due to disruption of one or more levels of the hypothalamic-pituitary-testicular axis.

Classification of hypogonadism [35]: Abnormalities of the hypothalamic-pituitary-testicular axis at the testicular level cause primary testicular failure, whereas central defects of the hypothalamus or pituitary cause secondary testicular failure. Hypogonadism also can reflect dual defects that affect both the testis and the pituitary. Primary testicular failure results in low testosterone levels, impairment of spermatogenesis, and elevated gonadotropin levels. Secondary testicular failure results in low testosterone levels, impairment of spermatogenesis, and low or low-normal gonadotropin levels. Combined primary and secondary testicular failure results in low testosterone levels, impairment of spermatogenesis, and variable gonadotropin levels, depending on whether primary or secondary testicular failure predominates [35].

Studies demonstrate both a significant decline in serum testosterone levels of about 1% per year after the age of 30 years and a prevalence of 30% of low serum testosterone in men over age 60 [36, 37]. This has significant implications in terms of cardiac health. Malkin et al. [36] demonstrated a 20.9% prevalence in men with coronary heart disease. The authors showed a substantial decrease in overall and vascular mortality with hypogonadism, highlighting the fact that androgen deficiency may be a part of the underlying pathophysiology of atherosclerotic disease in men (Fig. 11.2a and 11.2b).

Recent data confirms that lower serum testosterone levels are associated with significant morbidity and mortality [38]. These authors used a clinical database to identify men older than 40 years with repeated testosterone levels obtained from October 1, 1994, to December 31, 1999, and without diagnosed prostate cancer. A low testosterone level was a total testosterone level of less than 250 ng/dL (<8.7 nmol/L) or a free testosterone level of less than 0.75 ng/dL (<0.03 nmol/L). Men were classified as having a low testosterone level (166 (19.3%)), an equivocal testosterone level (equal number of low and normal levels) (240 (28.0%)), or a normal testosterone level (452 (52.7%)). The risk for all-cause mortality was estimated using Cox proportional hazards regression models, adjusting for demographic and clinical covariates over a follow-up of up to 8 years. There were 452 men (52.7%) with normal testosterone levels, 240 (28.0%) with equivocal levels, and 166 (19.3%) with low levels. Testosterone levels differed significantly between the three groups (Fig. 11.3). Men with low testosterone levels were older, had a greater BMI, and had a greater prevalence of diabetes mellitus compared with men with normal testosterone levels. Men with equivocal testosterone levels had a greater BMI than men with normal testosterone levels. Men with low and normal testosterone levels had more testosterone levels obtained than men with equivocal testosterone levels. There were no significant differences between the groups in marital status; medical morbidity; prevalence of chronic obstructive pulmonary disease, human immunodeficiency virus, CAD, or hyperlipidemia; and treatment with opiates and glucocorticoids.

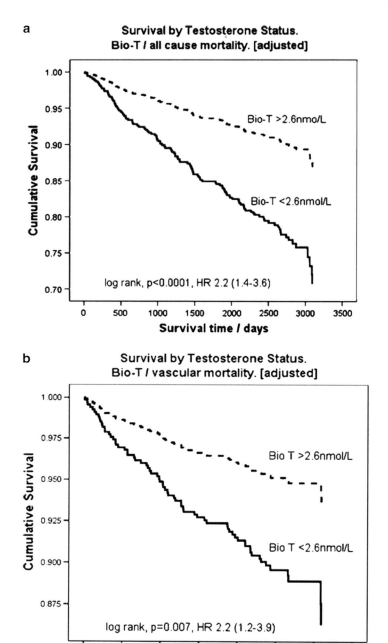

Fig. 11.2 Shows a survival curve of (**a**) all-cause mortality and (**b**) vascular mortality based on baseline bio-available testosterone (bio-T). The solid line represents patients with baseline bio-T less than 2.6 nmol/l, the broken line represents patients with bio-T greater than 2.6 nmol/l. HR, hazard ratio (from Malkin et al [36])

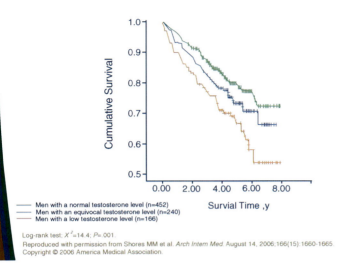

Low Testosterone Levels Associated With Increased Mortality Rate

Men with a normal testosterone level (n=452)
Men with an equivocal testosterone level (n=240)
Men with a low testosterone level (n=166)

Log-rank test; X^2=14.4; P=.001.
Reproduced with permission from Shores MM et al. *Arch Intern Med.* August 14, 2006;166(15):1660-1665.
Copyright © 2006 America Medical Association.

Fig. 11.3 A study was conducted to determine whether low testosterone levels are a risk factor for mortality in men 40 years of age or older. From the clinical database at the Veterans Affairs Puget Sound Health Care System, 858 male veterans who had repeated measurement of testosterone levels and no history of prostate or testicular cancer or antiandrogen treatment were identified. Testosterone levels were categorized as low if total testosterone was <250 ng/dL or free testosterone was <0.75 ng/dL. Testosterone levels were low in 166 men (19.3%), equivocal (equal number of low and normal levels) in 240 men (28%), and normal in 452 men (52.7%). Cox proportional hazards regression models, adjusted for demographic and clinical covariates over an 8-year follow-up period, were used to compare differences in survival times between men with low, equivocal, and normal testosterone levels. As illustrated by the Kaplan-Meier survival analysis, survival times were shorter in men with low or equivocal testosterone levels than in those with normal testosterone levels. All-cause mortality was 34.9% in men with low testosterone levels, 24.6% in men with equivocal testosterone levels, and 20.1% in men with normal testosterone levels (from Shores et al. [38])

The data demonstrated that mortality in men with normal testosterone levels was 20.1% (95% confidence interval (CI), 16.2%–24.1%) vs. 24.6% (95% CI, 19.2%–30.0%) in men with equivocal testosterone levels and 34.9% (95% CI, 28.5%–41.4%) in men with low testosterone levels. After adjusting for age, medical morbidity, and other clinical covariates, low testosterone levels continued to be associated with increased mortality (hazard ratio, 1.88; 95% CI, 1.34–2.63; P<0.001) while equivocal testosterone levels were not significantly different from normal testosterone levels (hazard ratio, 1.38; 95% CI, 0.99%–1.92%; P=0.06).

A decline in serum testosterone in the aging male may be directly associated with a loss of sexual desire and erectile dysfunction [39, 40]. The authors in the EMAS study group [39] surveyed a random population sample of 3,369 men between the ages of 40 and 79 years at eight European centers. Using question-naires, they collected data with regard to the subjects' general, sexual, physical, and psychological health. Levels of total testosterone were measured in morning blood samples by mass spectrometry, and free testosterone levels were calculated with the use of Vermeulen's formula. Data were randomly split into separate training and validation sets for confirmatory analyses.

In the training set, symptoms of poor morning erection, low sexual desire, erec-tile dysfunction, inability to perform vigorous activity, depression, and fatigue were significantly related to the testosterone level. Increased probabilities of the three sexual symptoms and limited physical vigor were discernible with decreased testos-terone levels (ranges, 8.0–13.0 nmol/L (2.3 to 3.7 ng/mL) for total testosterone and 160–280 pmol/L (46–81 pg/mL) for free testosterone). However, only the three sexual symptoms had a syndromic association with decreased testosterone levels. An inverse relationship between an increasing number of sexual symptoms and a decreasing testosterone level was observed. These relationships were independently confirmed in the validation set, in which the strengths of the association between symptoms and low testosterone levels determined the minimum criteria necessary to identify late-onset hypogonadism. Thus, late-onset hypogonadism can be defined by the presence of at least three sexual symptoms associated with a total testoster-one level of less than 11 nmol/L (3.2 ng/mL) and a free testosterone level of less than 220 pmol/L (64 pg/mL).

Assessment of Sexual Dysfunction in Aging Men and Women

Sexual Medicine History and Physical Examination [41]

The office evaluation consists of a series of direct questions about the nature of the sexual dysfunction complaint, as delineated in Table 11.1 for the male with sexual dysfunction (adapted from [41]). The interview should take place in a quiet room, in a nonjudgmental fashion. These men and women are embarrassed and often need reassurance that this topic is acceptable to discuss. The questions should be asked in a gentle manner, avoiding any gestures or posturing that might be misconstrued. While, it is worthwhile to for the patient to bring his/her partner into the office for further history, queries, and discussion at the time of the visit, it should be recog-nized that this is very uncommon. A similar interview paradigm should be employed for the female patient with sexual dysfunction [42].

Suggested laboratory work for the male patient presenting with sexual dysfunc-tion is offered in Table 11.2 [41]. Clinician judgment is used here. For example, if the patient is a known diabetic, a serum glucose many not be needed. Thus, these tests are obtained based upon the clinical scenario.

The objective assessment of male and female sexual function has been challeng-ing. Most regulatory agencies have allowed self-reported, validated instruments to be used as surrogate markers for sexual activity endpoints. Many instruments have

Table 11.1 Office evaluation questions for sexual dysfunction in aging men (from [41])

Characterize the sexual dysfunction

What type of sexual problem does the patient complain of?

For the male

Does he have ED, low desire, premature ejaculation, and delayed ejaculation?

If so, how long has he had the problem?

When was the last time he had intercourse?

When was the last time he had any sexual activity?

Does the sexual problem bother him?

Does the sexual problem bother his partner?

Did the problem arise suddenly (psychogenic), or has it arisen gradually?

Did the problem start when he started a new medication?

Does the problem occur with his partner only, or does it also occur without his partner, for example, with masturbation?

Does the problem occur because he has no partner or an uninterested partner?

Does he have a partner outside of his main relationship?

Can he get an erection? If so, is it firm enough for penetration?

Can he maintain the erection for intercourse?

Does he have a problem with sexual desire?

How long has he lost sexual desire?

Has he lost sexual desire with all partners?

Has he lost desire under all circumstances?

Has he lost desire because he cannot get or maintain an erection?

Has he lost desire because his partner has lost desire?

Does the patient complain of other associated symptoms, such as being tired, loss of stamina, loss of strength, loss of muscle mass, loss of muscle tone, recent weight gain, fatigue, or sleep issues?

Is the patient depressed?

Does he have a problem with ejaculation?

What type of ejaculation problem does the patient complain of?

When did the problem start?

Is the problem bothersome to the patient?

Is the problem bothersome to the partner?

Does the problem occur under all circumstances?

been published that meet or fulfill these needs. It is important to bear in mind that to our knowledge, these instruments are not specific to the aging male or female population, but rather are for general use. Data for the aging male and female is extrapolated from these instruments.

The instrument that has been used most often used to capture the severity of general male sexual function, and male erectile function in specific is the International Index of Erectile Function (IIEF, Table 11.3). This instrument was developed as an adjunctive sexual function measure for the sildenafil clinical trials [43] and has since gained universal acceptance as the leading instrument to assess male erectile function. A five question–shorter form was subsequently developed, which has been utilized quite widely as well ([44], Table 11.4). The IIEF and its shorter version have been used for all the clinical phosphodiesterase type 5 (PDE5) inhibitor trials along

Table 11.2 Common laboratory work for a man complaining
of sexual dysfunction, ED in particular (from [41])

Fasting lipid profile
Fasting glucose
TT and FT (morning testing preferred)
PSA: mandatory if considering testosterone supplementation; otherwise, it may be optional
Optional laboratory tests
Prolactin
Creatinine
Estradiol
Thyroid-stimulating hormone (TSH)
Follicle-stimulating hormone (FSH)
Luteinizing hormone (LH)
Dehydroepiandrosterone (DHEA)
25-hydroxyvitamin D level
SHBG
Albumin
Urinalysis

with numerous non-pharma-sponsored trials. The IIEF contains 15 questions which ask the patient to recall sexual activity for the previous 4 weeks. The 15 questions are answered on a Likert-type scale which allows the instrument to be graded numerically. Questions 1–5 and 15 are termed the erectile function domain of the IIEF.

Male ejaculatory function may be assessed by a variety of instruments. A recent, noteworthy instrument is the Male Sexual Health Questionnaire, which has been shortened to a 4-question instrument ([45], Table 11.5 and Table 11.6).

Testosterone deficiency in the male can be assessed by a variety of instruments. The Androgen Deficiency in the Aging Male (ADAM) questionnaire is widely used but unfortunately is not validated [46]. Further, the ADAM questionnaire (Table 11.7) seems to be sensitive but not specific for the diagnosis of hypogonadism. An answer of YES to questions 1 or 7 or any 3 other questions, suggest that the patient may be experiencing androgen deficiency (low testosterone level). The Aging Males' Symptom (AMS) questionnaire is often utilized as well [47]. Recently, the NERI hypogonadism screener has been published, but has not yet found its way into routine clinical practice [48].

The Centers for Epidemiologic Study–Depression scale is a public domain, user-friendly instrument to assess depressive symptoms [49]. It is easily interpreted and its use encouraged (Table 11.8).

Female Sexual Function

There are several well-done, validated, instruments that assess female sexual function [50]. One such instrument that seems to be gaining in popularity is the FSFI.

Table 11.3 IIEF questionnaire

Instructions: These questions ask about the effects your erection problems have had on your sex life, over the past 4 weeks. Please answer the following questions as honestly and clearly as possible. In answering these questions, the following definitions apply:

Definitions: Sexual activity includes intercourse, caressing, foreplay, and masturbation. Sexual intercourse is defined as vaginal penetration of the partner (you entered the partner). Sexual stimulation includes situations like foreplay with a partner, looking at erotic pictures, etc. Ejaculate is defined as the ejection of semen from the penis (or the feeling of this)

Mark ONLY one circle per question

1. Over the past 4 weeks, how often were you able to get an erection during sexual activity?
   0 No sexual activity
   0 Almost always or always
   0 Most times (much more than half the time)
   0 Sometimes (about half the time)
   0 A few times (much less than half the time)
   0 Almost never or never

2. Over the past 4 weeks, when you had erections with sexual stimulation, how often were your erections hard enough for penetration?
   0 No sexual stimulation
   0 Almost always or always
   0 Most times (much more than half the time)
   0 Sometimes (about half the time)
   0 A few times (much less than half the time)
   0 Almost never or never

Questions 3, 4, and 5 will ask about erections you may have had during sexual intercourse.

3. Over the past 4 weeks, when you attempted sexual intercourse, how often were you able to penetrate (enter) your partner?
   0 Did not attempt intercourse
   0 Almost always or always
   0 Most times (much more than half the time)
   0 Sometimes (about half the time)
   0 A few times (much less than half the time)
   0 Almost never or never

4. Over the past 4 weeks, during sexual intercourse, how often were you able to maintain your erection after you had penetrated (entered) your partner?
   0 Did not attempt intercourse
   0 Almost always or always
   0 Most times (much more than half the time)
   0 Sometimes (about half the time)
   0 A few times (much less than half the time)
   0 Almost never or never

5. Over the past 4 weeks, during sexual intercourse, how difficult was it to maintain your erection to completion of intercourse?
   0 Did not attempt intercourse
   0 Almost always or always
   0 Most times (much more than half the time)
   0 Sometimes (about half the time)
   0 A few times (much less than half the time)
   0 Almost never or never

(continued)

Table 11.3 (continued)

6. Over the past 4 weeks, how many times have you attempted sexual intercourse?
  0 No attempts
  0 1–2 attempts
  0 3–4 attempts
  0 5–6 attempts
  0 7–10 attempts
  0 11 or more attempts
7. Over the past 4 weeks, when you attempted sexual intercourse how often was it satisfactory for you?
  0 Did not attempt intercourse
  0 Almost always or always
  0 Most times (much more than half the time)
  0 Sometimes (about half the time)
  0 A few times (much less than half the time)
  0 Almost never or never
8. Over the past 4 weeks, how much have you enjoyed sexual intercourse?
  0 No intercourse
  0 Very highly enjoyable
  0 Highly enjoyable
  0 Fairly enjoyable
  0 Not very enjoyable
  0 Not enjoyable
9. Over the past 4 weeks, when you had sexual stimulation or intercourse how often did you ejaculate?
  0 Did not attempt intercourse
  0 Almost always or always
  0 Most times (more than half the time)
  0 Sometimes (about half the time)
  0 A few times (much less than half the time)
  0 Almost never or never
10. Over the past 4 weeks, when you had sexual stimulation or intercourse how often did you have the feeling of orgasm or climax (with or without ejaculation)?
  0 No sexual stimulation or intercourse
  0 Almost always or always
  0 Most times (much more than half the time)
  0 Sometimes (about half the time)
  0 A few times (much less than half the time)
  0 Almost never or never
Questions 11 and 12 ask about sexual desire. Let's define sexual desire as a feeling that may include wanting to have a sexual experience (for example, masturbation or intercourse), thinking about having sex or feeling frustrated due to lack of sex
11. Over the past 4 weeks, how often have you felt sexual desire?
  0 Almost always or always
  0 Most times (much more than half the time)
  0 Sometimes (about half the time)
  0 A few times (much less than half the time)
  0 Almost never or never

(continued)

Table 11.3 (continued)

12. Over the past 4 weeks, how would you rate your level of sexual desire?
    0 Very high
    0 High
    0 Moderate
    0 Low
    0 Very low or none at all
13. Over the past 4 weeks, how satisfied have you been with you overall sex life?
    0 Very satisfied
    0 Moderately satisfied
    0 About equally satisfied and dissatisfied
    0 Moderately dissatisfied
    0 Very dissatisfied
14. Over the past 4 weeks, how satisfied have you been with your sexual relationship with your partner?
    0 Very satisfied
    0 Moderately satisfied
    0 About equally satisfied and dissatisfied
    0 Moderately dissatisfied
    0 Very dissatisfied
15. Over the past 4 weeks, how do you rate your confidence that you can get and keep your *erection*?
    0 Very high
    0 High
    0 Moderate
    0 Low
    0 Very low

All items are scored in five domains as follows[a]:

Domain	Items	Range	Max score
Erectile function	1, 2, 3, 4, 5, 15	0–5	30
Orgasmic function	9, 10	0–5	10
Sexual desire	11, 12	0–5	10
Intercourse satisfaction	6, 7, 8	0–5	15
Overall satisfaction	13, 14	0-5	10

[a]Scoring algorithm for IIEF

The FSFI is a brief multidimensional scale for assessing sexual function in women. The scale has received psychometric evaluation, including studies of reliability, convergent validity, and discriminant validity. The authors' found an FSFI total score of 26.55 to be the optimal cut score for differentiating women with and without sexual dysfunction [51]. The FSFI has been recently validated for use in cancer survivors [52].

While this validated cutpoint for the total FSFI scale score of 26.55 enables one to classify women into groups with and without sexual dysfunction, there was no sexual desire (SD) domain-specific cutpoint for assessing the presence of diminished desire in women with or without a sexual desire problem. Gersterberger et al. noted that the use of a diagnostic cutpoint for classifying women with SD scores of

Table 11.4 The International Index of Erectile Function (IIEF-5) questionnaire (from Rosen et al. [44])

Over the past 6 months	Very low 1	Low 2	Moderate 3	High 4	Very high 5
1. How do you rate your *confidence* that you could get and keep an erection?	Very low 1	Low 2	Moderate 3	High 4	Very high 5
2. When you had erections with sexual stimulation, *how often* were your erections hard enough for penetration?	Almost never/ never 1	A few times (much less than half the time) 2	Sometimes (about half the time) 3	Most times (much more than half the time) 4	Almost always/ always 5
3. During sexual intercourse, *how often* were you able to maintain your erection after you had penetrated (entered) your partner?	Almost never/ never 1	A few times (much less than half the time) 2	Sometimes (about half the time) 3	Most times (much more than half the time)4	Almost always/ always 5
4. During sexual intercourse, *how difficult* was it to maintain your erection to completion of intercourse?	Extremely difficult 1	Very difficult 2	Difficult 3	Slightly difficult 4	Not difficult 5
5. When you attempted sexual intercourse, *how often* was it satisfactory for you?	Almost never/ never 1	A few times (much less than half the time) 2	Sometimes (about half the time) 3	Most times (much more than half the time) 4	Almost always/ always 5

IIEF-5 scoring:
The IIEF-5 score is the sum of the ordinal responses to the five items
22–25: No erectile dysfunction
17–21: Mild erectile dysfunction
12–16: Mild to moderate erectile dysfunction
8–11: Moderate erectile dysfunction
5–7: Severe erectile dysfunction

Table 11.5 Male sexual health questionnaire (MSHQ)

Erection scale*

1. *In the last month*, without using drugs like Viagra, how often have you been able to get an erection when you wanted to? (check only one)

    5 All of the time

    4 Most of the time

    3 About half of the time

    2 Less than half of the time

    1 None of the time

    0 Used Viagra or similar drug with every sexual encounter

2. In the last month, if you were able to get an erection, without using drugs like Viagra, how often were you able to stay hard as long as you wanted to? (check only one)

    5 All of the time

    4 Most of the time

    3 About half of the time

    2 Less than half of the time

    1 None of the time

    0 Used Viagra or similar drug with every sexual encounter

3. *In the last month*, if you were able to get an erection, without using drugs like Viagra, how would you rate the hardness of your erection? (check only one)

    5 Completely hard

    4 Almost completely hard

    3 Mostly hard, but can be slightly bent

    2 A little hard, but bends easily

    1 Not at all hard

    0 Used Viagra or similar drug with every sexual encounter

INTRODUCTION: The following questions concern various aspects of your ability to have sex. In answering these questions, please think about all aspects of the sexual activity you have had with your main partner, with other partners, or masturbating.

By sexual activity, we mean any type of sex you may have had, including intercourse, oral sex, or other sexual activities that could lead to ejaculation. Some of these questions might be difficult to answer. Please answer as many as possible, and be as honest as you can when answering them. Please remember that all of your answers are confidential. The first questions concern your erections, which some people refer to as "hard-one." In the last month have you taken Viagra or any similar drugs for problems with your erection? Yes No

ED Bother Item

4. *In the last month*, if you have had difficulty getting hard or staying hard without using drugs like Viagra, have you been bothered by this problem?… (Check only one)

    5 Not at all bothered/Did not have a problem with erection

    4 A little bit bothered

    3 Moderately bothered

    2 Very bothered

    1 Extremely bothered

Ejaculation (Ej) scale

INTRODUCTION: The next section deals with male ejaculation and the pleasure you have with ejaculation.

Ejaculation or "cumming" is the release of semen or "cum" during sexual climax. These questions concern all

(continued)

Table 11.5 (continued)

of your ejaculations when having sexual activity. These could include ejaculations you have had with your

main partner, as well as with other partners, or ejaculations you have had when masturbating.

5. *In the last month*, how often have you been able to ejaculate when having sexual activity? (check only one)

    5 All of the time

    4 Most of the time

    3 About half of the time

    2 Less than half of the time

    1 None of the time/could not ejaculate

6. *In the last month,* when having sexual activity, how often did you feel that you took too long to ejaculate or "cum"? (check only one)

    5 None of the time

    4 Less than half of the time

    3 About half of the time

    2 Most of the time

    1 All of the time

    0 Could not ejaculate

7. *In the last month*, when having sexual activity, how often have you felt like you were ejaculating ("cumming"), but no fluid came out?

    5 None of the time

    4 Less than half of the time

    3 About half of the time

    2 Most of the time

    1 All of the time

    0 Could not ejaculate

8. In the last month, how would you rate the strength or force of your ejaculation?

    5 As strong as it always was

    4 A little less strong than it used to be

    3 Somewhat less strong than it used to be

    2 Much less strong than it used to be

    1 Very much less strong than it used to be

    0 Could not ejaculate

9. *In the last month*, how would you rate the amount or volume of semen when you ejaculate?

    5 As much as it always was

    4 A little less than it used to be

    3 Somewhat less than it used to be

    2 Much less than it used to be

    1 Very much less than it used to be

    0 Could not ejaculate

10. *Compared to ONE month ago,* would you say the physical pleasure you feel when you ejaculate has…

    5 Increased a lot

    4 Increased moderately

    3 Neither increased nor decreased

    2 Decreased moderately

    1 Decreased a lot

    0 Could not ejaculate

(continued)

Table 11.5 (continued)

11. In the last month, have you experienced any physical pain or discomfort when you ejaculated? Would you say you have…

    5 No pain at all

    4 Slight amount of pain or discomfort

    3 Moderate amount of pain or discomfort

    2 Strong amount of pain or discomfort

    1 Extreme amount of pain or discomfort

    0 Could not ejaculate

(EjD) bother item

12. *In the last month,* if you have had any ejaculation difficulties or have been unable to ejaculate, have you been bothered by this?

    5 Not at all bothered

    4 A little bit bothered

    3 Moderately bothered

    2 Very bothered

    1 Extremely bothered

Satisfaction scale

These next few questions ask about your relationship with your main partner over the *last month.*

Some of these questions concern your sexual relationship, while others are about your overall relationship.

13. Generally, how satisfied are you with the overall sexual relationship you have with your main partner? (check only one)

    5 Extremely satisfied

    4 Moderately satisfied

    3 Neither satisfied nor unsatisfied

    2 Moderately unsatisfied

    1 Extremely unsatisfied

14. Generally, how satisfied are you with the quality of the sex life you have with your main partner?

    5 Extremely satisfied

    4 Moderately satisfied

    3 Neither satisfied nor unsatisfied

    2 Moderately unsatisfied

    1 Extremely unsatisfied

15. Generally, how satisfied are you with the number of times you and your main partner have sex?

    5 Extremely satisfied

    4 Moderately satisfied

    3 Neither satisfied nor unsatisfied

    2 Moderately unsatisfied

    1 Extremely unsatisfied

16. Generally, how satisfied are you with the way you and your main partner show affection during sex?

    5 Extremely satisfied

    4 Moderately satisfied

    3 Neither satisfied nor unsatisfied

    2 Moderately unsatisfied

    1 Extremely unsatisfied

(continued)

Table 11.5 (continued)

17. Generally, how satisfied are you with the way you and your main partner communicate about sex?

    5 Extremely satisfied

    4 Moderately satisfied

    3 Neither satisfied nor unsatisfied

    2 Moderately unsatisfied

    1 Extremely unsatisfied

18. Aside from your sexual relationship, how satisfied are you with all other aspects of the relationship you have with your main partner?

    5 Extremely satisfied

    4 Moderately satisfied

    3 Neither satisfied nor unsatisfied

    2 Moderately unsatisfied

    1 Extremely unsatisfied

Additional items (sexual activity and desire)

19. *In the last month*, how often have you had sexual activity, including masturbating, intercourse, oral sex, or any other type of sex? (check only one)

    5 Daily or almost daily

    4 More than 6 times per month

    3 4–6 times per month

    2 1–3 times per month

    1 0 times per month

If your answer is "0" for item 19, please answer the following questions:

A. When was the last time you had sex? (check only one)

    5 1–3 months ago

    4 4–6 months ago

    3 7–12 months ago

    2 13–24 months ago

    1 More than 24 months ago

B. What are the reasons you have not had sex?

I could not have sex because I could not get an erection: Yes No

I could not have sex because I could not ejaculate or "cum": Yes No

I had no partner:

Yes No

Other (specify): _____

20. Compared to *ONE month ago*, has the number of times you have had sexual activity increased or decreased?

    5 Increased a lot

    4 Increased moderately

    3 Neither increased nor decreased

    2 Decreased moderately

    1 Decreased a lot

INTRODUCTION: The next set of questions concern the sexual activity you have had *in the last month*. In answering these questions, we want to know about all of the sexual activity you have had with your main partner, with other partners, or masturbating. By sexual activity, we mean any type of sex you may have had, including intercourse, oral sex, or any other sexual activities that could lead to ejaculation.

(continued)

Table 11.5 (continued)

21. *In the last month*, have you been bothered by these changes in the number of times you have had sexual activity?

    5 Not at all bothered

    4 A little bit bothered

    3 Moderately bothered

    2 Very bothered

    1 Extremely bothered

INTRODUCTION: These next questions ask about your urge or desire to have sex with *your main partner*. Some people refer to this as "feeling horny." These questions concern the sexual urges you have felt toward your main partner, and not whether you actually had sex

Do you have a "main partner"? :

Yes No

IF YOU DO NOT HAVE A MAIN PARTNER, PLEASE ANSWER ALL QUESTIONS WITHOUT REFERENCE TO A "MAIN PARTNER"

22. *In the last month,* how often have you felt an urge or desire to have sex with your main partner?

    5 All of the time

    4 Most of the time

    3 About half of the time

    2 Less than half of the time

    1 None of the time

23. *In the last month,* how would you rate your urge or desire to have sex with your main partner?

    5 Very high

    4 High

    3 Moderate

    2 Low

    1 Very low or none at all

24. *In the last month*, have you been bothered by your level of sexual desire? Have you been…

    5 Not at all bothered

    4 A little bit bothered

    3 Moderately bothered

    2 Very bothered

    1 Extremely bothered

25. Compared to *ONE month ago,* has your urge or desire for sex with your main partner increased or decreased?

    5 Increased a lot

    4 Increased moderately

    3 Neither increased nor decreased

    2 Decreased moderately

    1 Decreased a lot

Thank You for Your Cooperation

*Courtesy of MAPI Research Trust

Table 11.6 MSHQ-EjD short form for assessing EjD*

In the past month:

1. How often have you been able to ejaculate or "cum" when having sexual activity?

All the time	5
Most of the time	4
About half the time	3
Less than half the time	2
None of the time/could not ejaculate	1

2. How would you rate the strength or force of your ejaculation?

As strong as it always was	5
A little less strong than it used to be	4
Somewhat less strong than it used to be	3
Much less strong than it used to be	2
Very much less strong than it used to be	1
Could not ejaculate	0

3. How would you rate the amount or volume of semen or fluid when you ejaculate?

As much as it always was	5
A little less than it used to be	4
Somewhat less than it used to be	3
Much less than it used to be	2
Very much less than it used to be	1
Could not ejaculate	0

4. If you have had any ejaculation difficulties or have been unable to ejaculate, have you been bothered by this?

No problem with ejaculation	0
Not at all bothered	1
A little bothered	2
Moderately bothered	3
Very bothered	4
Extremely bothered	5

*Courtesy of MAPI Research Trust

5 or less on the SD domain of the FSFI as having HSDD and those with SD scores of 6 or more as not having HSDD maximized diagnostic sensitivity and specificity. In the development sample, the sensitivity and specificity for predicting HSDD (with or without other conditions) were 75% and 84%, respectively, and the corresponding sensitivity and specificity in the validation sample were 92% and 89%, respectively [53].

Table 11.7 Saint Louis University

Adam questionnaire*

Androgen deficiency in aging males

1. Do you have a decrease in libido (sex drive)?
2. Do you have a lack of energy?
3. Do you have a decrease in strength and/or endurance?
4. Have you lost height?
5. Have you noticed a decreased "enjoyment of life"?
6. Are you sad and/or grumpy?
7. Are your erections less strong?
8. Have you noted a recent deterioration in your ability to play sports?
9. Are you falling asleep after dinner?
10. Has there been a recent deterioration in your work performance?

*This questionnaire was developed by John E. Morley, M.B., B.Ch. It is to be used solely as a screening tool to assist your physician in diagnosing androgen deficiency

Table 11.8 Center for Epidemiologic Studies Depression Scale (CES-D), NIMH

SAINT LOUIS UNIVERSITY

ADAM QUESTIONNAIRE

ANDROGEN DEFICIENCY IN AGING MALES

1. Do you have a decrease in libido (sex drive)? _____
2. Do you have a lack of energy? _____
3. Do you have a decrease in strength and/or endurance? _____
4. Have you lost height? _____
5. Have you noticed a decreased "enjoyment of life"? _____
6. Are you sad and/or grumpy? _____
7. Are your erections less strong? _____
8. Have you noted a recent deterioration in your ability to play sports? _____
9. Are you falling asleep after dinner? _____
10. Has there been a recent deterioration in your work performance? _____

This questionnaire was developed by John E. Morley, M.B., B.Ch. It is to be used solely as a screening tool to assist your physician in diagnosing androgen deficiency.

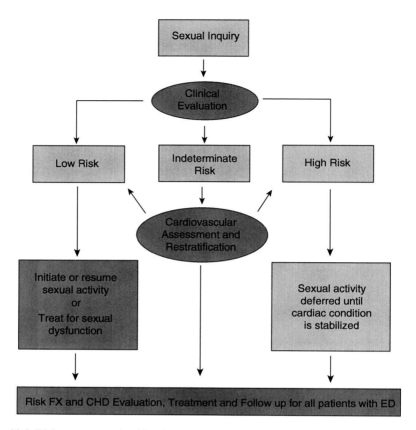

Fig. 11.4 Risk assessment algorithm for men with cardiovascular risk factors who wish to reengage in sexual activity (from Kostis et al. [54])

It is important to recognize that many clinicians find these questionnaires somewhat cumbersome to use during the office visit. Rather than using the full instrument, clinicians have adopted their practices so that they utilize a modified version of a specific instrument. This seems to suit them well.

There are many other wonderful instruments that have been developed to assess male and female sexual function. The authors of these fine instruments deserve recognition and we offer our apologies for our inability to include them and credit them in this section. Finally, there are many instruments that evaluate mood, depression, cognition, strength, quality of life, amongst other areas, in the aging male and female. Discussion of these instruments is beyond the scope of this chapter.

Cardiovascular evaluation of the male and female patient with sexual dysfunction: Consensus guidelines have provided algorithms to the clinician as to which patients with cardiovascular risk factors may safely reengage in sexual activity. The Princeton II consensus guidelines document discusses the approach for men with a variety of CV risk factors and their ability to reengage in sexual activity ([54], Fig. 11.4). Low risk patients are those with less than three CV risk factors, controlled hypertension, etc. The reader should review ref [54] to gain a better understanding of the risk assessment algorithm. The Princeton III conference was recently convened to continue the discussion of evaluating CV risks and sexual health [55]. Importantly, data from that meeting has surfaced that reviews CV risk and female sexual health [56]. Other, recent guidelines have been offered to assist the clinician with counseling patients who have various CV issues and wish to reengage in sexual activity [57].

Pathophysiology of ED

This area has studied in depth and thus data on erectile dysfunction (ED) is well-represented in the literature. Erectile dysfunction is defined as the consistent inability to achieve or maintain an erection adequate for satisfactory sexual function [58]. Age alone is the single most profound variable associated with erectile dysfunction and impotence. Feldman et al. showed that the rate of complete impotence tripled from 5 to 15% as men aged from the 40 to 70 [28]. After adjustment for age, a higher probability of ED was directly correlated with cardiovascular disease, hypertension, diabetes mellitus (DM), and depression, and inversely correlated with serum dehydroepiandrosterone (DHEA), high density lipoprotein cholesterol and an index of dominant personality. ED can significantly decrease the quality of life as well as a man's mental and physical wellbeing. The cause of ED is primarily organic but can have a psychogenic etiology as well [28, 41].

ED can be caused by endocrine abnormalities, most commonly DM, but also hypogonadism and hyperprolactinemia [41, 59, 60]. DM causes changes in neurotransmitters like nitric oxide and vasoactive intestinal peptide resulting in poor erectile ability; tight glycemic control has been shown to dramatically reduce the prevalence of ED (Fig. 11.5, [61–63]). Complications of smooth muscle and endothelial dysfunction are sequelae of DM, which can exacerbate the severity of ED by direct pathophysiology.

Vascular and hypertensive disease can worsen the severity of ED and bring an earlier onset of impotence. The primary mechanisms are arterial insufficiency and venous leakage. Atherosclerosis leads to arterial occlusive disease, which can decrease the perfusion pressure and arterial flow to the lacunar spaces necessary for penile rigidity. Subsequently, adequate pressure is not achieved within the corpora cavernosa because of excessive venous outflow through the subtunical venules and thus no erection occurs [62, 63].

Other causes include neurologic deficits such as cerebrovascular accidents (CVA), Parkinson's disease, multiple sclerosis, and spinal cord injury. Direct injury to the penis itself either by trauma or by other pathologies like priapism can contribute to varying degrees of ED. Finally there are several psychogenic causes such as anxiety, depression, and stress-related issues that decrease the strength and duration of an erection or outright prevent initiation of the erection (Table 11.9, [61]).

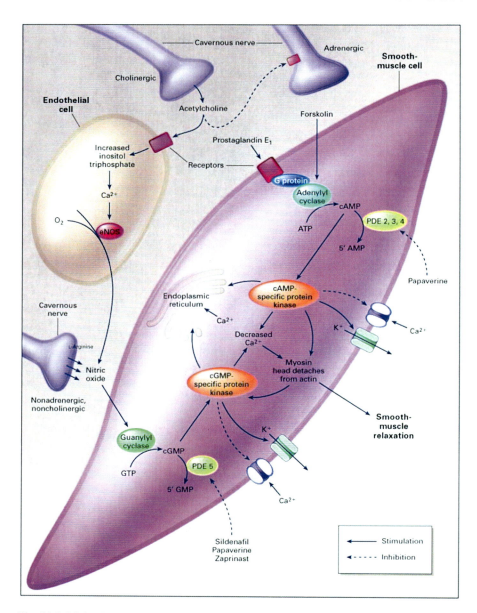

Fig. 11.5 Molecular mechanism of penile smooth-muscle relaxation. Cyclic AMP (cAMP) and cyclic GMP (cGMP), the intracellular second messengers mediating smooth-muscle relaxation, activate their specific protein kinases, which phosphorylate certain proteins to cause opening of potassium channels, closing of calcium channels, and sequestration of intracellular calcium by the endoplasmic reticulum. The resultant fall in intracellular calcium leads to smooth-muscle relaxation. Sildenafil inhibits the action of phosphodiesterase (PDE) type 5, thus increasing the intracellular concentration of cGMP. Papaverine is a nonspecific phosphodiesterase inhibitor. GTP denotes guanosine triphosphate and eNOS endothelial nitric oxide synthase. (from Lue [61])

Table 11.9 Classification and common causes of erectile dysfunction (from [61])

Category of erectile dysfunction	Common disorders	Pathophysiology
Psychogenic	Performance anxiety Relationship problems Psychological stress Depression	Loss of libido, over inhibition, or impaired nitric oxide release
Neurogenic	Stroke or Alzheimer's disease Spinal cord injury Radical pelvic surgery Diabetic neuropathy Pelvic injury	Failure to initiate nerve impulse or interrupted neural transmission
Hormonal	Hypogonadism Hyperprolactinemia	Loss of libido and inadequate nitric oxide release
Vasculogenic (arterial or cavernosal)	Atherosclerosis Hypertension Diabetes mellitus Trauma Peyronie's disease	Inadequate arterial flow or impaired venoocclusion
Drug-induced	Antihypertensive and antidepressant drugs	Central suppression
	Antiandrogens	Decreased libido
	Alcohol abuse	Alcoholic neuropathy
	Cigarette smoking	Vascular insufficiency
Caused by other systemic diseases and aging	Old age	Usually multifactorial, resulting in neural and vascular dysfunction

Although the clinical presentation of ED is the same, the diagnosis requires a complete history and a basic genital examination, especially looking for Peyronie's plaque and femoral bruits, evaluating secondary sexual characteristics, and general physical exam including blood pressure assessment. Laboratory values of blood glucose, cholesterol, and testosterone levels usually supplement an evaluation [41].

Pathophysiology of the Role of Hypogonadism in Sexual Dysfunction in the Aging Male

The effects of hypogonadism on male sexual desire seem to be well established [64]. The true contribution of hypogonadism to erectile and ejaculatory function is the subject of intense debate. It postulated that penile erectile tissue possesses high concentrations of locally synthesized androgens and that testosterone-dependent functions are not a reflection of circulating androgen levels [65]. In several animal studies, testosterone deprivation changed the response and structural functionality of erectile tissue [66]. Testosterone is required for adequate function of nitric oxide synthase, which produces nitric oxide necessary for relaxation of cavernosal endothelial and corporeal smooth muscle resulting in erection [67]. Penile erection can also be mediated through a non-nitric oxide-dependent pathway with the stimulation of cyclic AMP synthesis [61, 68]. Testosterone has also been shown to inhibit detrusor muscle contractions and thus lower testosterone levels may contribute to unstable function of the detrusor muscle and lower urinary tract symptoms (LUTS), especially in men with BPH [69].

Lower levels of testosterone also play a significant role in decreasing muscle mass, increasing fat mass, and weaker bone density as men age. Free testosterone has been shown to be the best predictor of loss of muscle mass and strength in the New Mexico Aging Process Study [70]. Sarcopenia eventually leads to frailty and subsequent functional deterioration as well as a substantial decrease in sexual functioning. Objectively, this is measured by unintentional weight loss, exhaustion and fatigue, general muscle weakness, and lower sexual appetite. In additional to androgen, other factors including age, caloric intake, and physical activity all play different roles in the pathophysiology of frailty and decreased sexual functionality [71]. In longitudinal studies, the combination of loss of hormones such as testosterone and insulin-like growth factors (IGF-1) and increase in cytokines like tumor necrosis factor (TNF-alpha) and interleukins (IL-6) provide the mechanism for the lost muscle mass and strength [72]. There is a direct effect of testosterone on osteoblasts contributing to increased bone mineral density [73]. However, the exact interactions between these hormones and their receptor activity and how further pathways contribute to muscle decline and higher rates of hip fractures are not well understood.

With respect to hypogonadism, decreased energy levels and impaired sexual performance were the two most important quality-of-life issues for older men in a recent study [74]. Dacal et al. demonstrated that lowering testosterone medically in patients with prostate cancer on androgen deprivation resulted in a large deterioration of quality of life. This encompasses not only the lower physical and sexual activity in older adults, but also poorer cognition, less coordination, and satisfaction with functionality [74].

Lower testosterone has been correlated with more severe atherosclerotic changes and increased intima media thickness [76, 77]. Low-dose supplemental testosterone has been shown to decrease the incidence of exercise-induced myocardial infarction and ST depression in men with chronic stable angina [78, 79]. It can be inferred from these studies that testosterone may contribute to a beneficial effect on the cardiovascular system.

Yet, in spite of these data, a recent meta-analysis conducted on behalf of the Agency for Healthcare Research and Quality, revealed that the efficacy of hormonal treatments and the value of hormone testing in men with ED were inconclusive [80].

Table 11.10 Specialized urologic and radiologic tests for men with erectile dysfunction (from [61])

Test	Indications
Combined penile injection of a vasodilator and sexual stimulation	Assess penile vascular function
	Therapeutic test in men who choose intracavernous therapy
Duplex (color) ultrasonography	Assess vascular function and evaluate for Peyronie's disease
Cavernosography	Young men with congenital or traumatic venous leakage
Pelvic arteriography	Young men with traumatic arterial insufficiency
Nocturnal penile monitoring (RigiScan ambulatory rigidity and Tumescence system, Timm medical, Minneapolis)	Differentiate psychogenic from organic erectile dysfunction

Testing for Erectile Dysfunction in the Aging Male

The paradigm has shifted in the field of male ED, and specifically ED in the aging male, such that the presumptive diagnosis is that the disease is either partly or fully organic in etiology. Historical tests to assess nocturnal erections, such as the snap-gauge and nocturnal penile tumescence testing have fallen by the wayside and are no longer used by most clinicians. Penile duplex Doppler ultrasound is used in conjunction with a penile injection of a vasoactive agent to induce an erection. This test is performed by select clinicians (urologists and/or radiologists) to assess the penile arterial tree and the penile capacity to trap blood under conditions that mimic an erection. Other tests are available as well (Table 11.10), and are utilized for select patients. In light of the fact that most clinicians and patients move forward with oral treatment of their ED irrespective of the etiology of the ED, the utility of these tests for the older male with ED is questioned. Nonetheless, the penile duplex Doppler is quite helpful in defining the cause of the ED when used under the appropriate conditions [81].

Thus, the diagnosis of male erectile dysfunction is made predominately on the history, with confirmatory testing limited to specific patients.

Testing for hypogonadism should be relatively simple. The diagnosis is made based upon the presence of symptoms, such as low libido, fatigue, and erectile dysfunction, combined with a serum testosterone of less than 300 ng/dL [82]. Mass screening of the population for low T is discouraged. While at face value this diagnosis should be relatively straightforward, the entire disease state, including the diagnosis has been the subject of recent debate. The assay to diagnose low has been scrutinized and is under intense review [83]. As it stands now, many of the assays in current use may fall by the wayside. Next, the lower level of normal, 300 ng/dL, has been discussed in depth and is not universally accepted [84]. Currently, many commercial labs have lower thresholds, e.g., 200 ng/dL, 242 ng/dL, 262 ng/dL, adding confusion to the mix. Additionally, there has been discussion that hypogonadism in older men, say over 65, is a distinct disease state, dissimilar to hypogonadism in younger men [39, 84]. While there are many advocates supporting the position that hypogonadism is highly prevalent in this older age group [84], others suggest that the actual incidence is quite low [39]. Thus, controversy abounds in this field. Adding further fuel to the fire, the Institute of Medicine published a very thorough review of this topic and offered the following in 2003, "Hypogonadism occurs in men of various ages, and most clinical studies of the therapy so far have been in younger hypogonadal men. Less is known about the potential beneficial or adverse effects of testosterone therapy in older males and there have been concerns regarding prostate outcomes" [85].

The diagnosis of ejaculatory dysfunction in the male is based upon history. The questionnaires mentioned above [43–45] may be as well. Rapid ejaculation and delayed ejaculation remain challenging areas for the clinician.

The diagnosis of FSD is made based upon history. Questionnaires are available to corroborate the diagnosis of HSDD [49–51]. There are no currently available FDA-approved treatment options for HSDD, adding challenges to this disease state. Flibanserin (Boehringer Ingelheim), an oral, dual 5-HT1A receptor agonist and 5-HT2A receptor antagonist, was not approved by the FDA recently for the treatment of HSDD in women [86]. The meaning and definition of low serum testosterone levels in women is a challenging area [87]. Normal serum levels of testosterone are not well established [88], and there is no currently available FDA-approved treatment for women with low testosterone. Intrinsa (Procter & Gamble), a testosterone patch for women was not approved by the FDA in 2004 [89]. Libigel (Biosante), a testosterone gel for women, failed to meet its study endpoints (2011) and thus will most likely not reach the marketplace [90] ERT in postmenospausal or surgically menopausal women has fallen into disfavor based upon cardiovascular and other evidence present by the WHI reports [22, 91, 92]. Findings from the Women's Health Initiative (WHI) Estrogen-Alone (E-Alone) trial were published in April 2004. The National Institutes of Health decided to stop this trial early because of an increased risk of stroke and no heart disease benefit in participants assigned to active estrogen pills compared to those assigned to placebo (inactive pills). The E-Alone trial included 10,739 postmenopausal women who were 50–79 years old and already had a hysterectomy when they joined the WHI. In the E-Alone trial, 5,310 women were assigned to take active conjugated equine estrogen pills (CEE or Premarin®) at a dosage of 0.625 mg each day and 5,429 were assigned to take placebo. The major findings from the trial were that E-alone increased the risk of strokes and blood clots in the legs, decreased the risk of hip fractures, and had no clear effect on heart disease or breast cancer.

For breast cancer, these initial findings suggested that women in the active estrogen (CEE) group had a 23% lower risk of breast cancer compared to those in the placebo group over an average follow-up of 6.8 years. While this difference was not statistically significant, the findings were viewed as surprising, because a significant increase in breast cancer risk was found in the other WHI hormone trial of combined estrogen plus progestin (E + P) in women who had a uterus when they joined the WHI. In the initial E-Alone report, limited data were published from the 218 invasive breast cancers that had been reported [91]. In April, 2006, the Journal of the American Medical Association published the final report of all breast cancers diagnosed before the E-Alone trial was stopped [92]. This report covered an average of 7.1 years of follow-up and analyzed detailed information from all 237 invasive breast cancers that occurred during the trial. Participants in the CEE group had a 20% lower risk of invasive breast cancer compared to those in the placebo group, similar to the findings in the initial report.

Detailed analyses showed no evidence that breast cancer risk shifted during the average 7 years of follow-up in the E-Alone trial. In contrast, in the E + P trial, the increase in risk of breast cancer emerged after 4 years.

Based on all of aforementioned issues, some authorities advocate the use topical estrogen (and testosterone) therapy in postmenopausal or surgically menopausal women, in lieu of the oral preparations [93]. This remains a controversial area.

Treatment of FSD in the aging female: Based upon the discussion presented above, there are concerns regarding hormonal replacement therapies for women with hormonally based sexual dysfunction, though there are proponents of topical hormonal replacement therapies. Oral therapy for HSDD was not approved by the FDA as noted above.

There are a group of women who have urinary incontinence and sexual dysfunction. Surgical or medical correction of the incontinence seems to improve the sexual issues [94, 95]. This is an underappreciated area of medical need for older women interested in restoration of sexual function.

As an example, one hundred fifty-seven women complaining of urodynamic stress incontinence underwent a mid-urethral sling (MUS) procedure [95]. All patients answered the Italian translation of FSFI, before and 12 months after surgery. Also included in the final analysis were all the women who are nonsexually active at baseline. The authors evaluated the prevalence of FSD according to the FSFI cutoff point (26.55).

One hundred thirty-three patients completed the study protocol: 105 out of 133 underwent a *trans*-obturator procedure, while 28 out of 133 had a retropubic procedure. After the 12-month follow-up, 115 out of 133 patients (86%) were dry, ten improved their symptoms, and the remaining eight were unchanged. Seventy-nine out of 133 (59%) patients reported an active sexual life before surgery. Fifty-four (41%) reported they were not sexually active before surgery. Twelve months after surgery, 22 out of 54 nonsexually active women (40%) reestablished sexual activity, whereas only 6 out of 79 (7.5%) patients, sexually active at baseline, were not sexually active 1 year after surgery ($P < 0.05$). After adjusting for multiple testing, only age, menopause, and storage symptoms remained significantly correlated with the FSFI total score postsurgery as independent variables. These data showed that after an MUS procedure, female sexual function improves. Interestingly, a very relevant percentage of nonsexually active women reported renewed sexual activity after MUS.

Treatment of Erectile Dysfunction in the Aging Male

There are many treatments for male ED including oral pills, injection of vasoactive agents into the corpus cavernosum, vacuum device therapies, intraurethral therapies, and surgical options [41, 61]. Oral therapies include the phosphodiesterase-5 inhibitor (PDE5-I) class of medications (sildenafil, vardenafil, and tadalafil). PDE5 is found in trabecular smooth muscle and it catalyzes the degradation of cGMP, which elevates cytoplasmic calcium concentrations leading to smooth muscle contraction. PDE5 inhibitors block this mechanism for improvement in erectile function [61, 96]. These classes of medication can substantially and rapidly decrease blood pressure in patients who are concurrently taking nitrates and are therefore contraindicated in patients taking any form of nitrate therapy. Historically, the PDE5-I have been taken orally, as on demand medications. Meaning, the oral drug was taken in proximity to the planned sexual event. Tadalafil provides a 36-h activity window while the other two drugs in the class indicate 4–8 h therapeutic windows. There are ample short-term data which support the safety and efficacy of tadalafil [97]. In general, these drugs are well tolerated and provide benefit to the majority of men who take them. Most men (50–80%) will see an improvement in their erectile function. Data, primarily from short-term trials (<or = 12 weeks), indicate that PDE-5 inhibitors were more effective than placebo in improving sexual intercourse success (69.0% vs. 35.0%). The proportion of men with improved erections was significantly greater among those treated with PDE-5 inhibitors (range, 67.0–89.0%) than with placebo (range, 27.0–35.0%) [74]. Interestingly, improvements in erectile function are gauged, in some studies, by an improvement in the IIEF score, among several other questionnaires [61, 80, 96, 97]. The improvement in erectile function will be proportional to dose of the drug taken. Data suggest that many men drop out of therapy approximately 1 year after starting therapy. It is unclear if this is due to drug cost (as many insurance plans do not cover this oral therapy), side effects, lack of efficacy, partner issues, or combinations thereof [98]. Side effects are mild, limited, well tolerated and usually do not cause the patient to cease therapy. The most common side effects include headache, rhinitis, dyspepsia, facial flushing, myalgia, and back pain [61, 80].

Specific data regarding the efficacy and safety of PDE5-I in older men is limited. The efficacy and safety of oral sildenafil (VIAGRA) for treating ED in elderly men (aged > or = 65 years or older) was reported in a 2002 review and a 2005 review [99, 100]. In the 2005 review, the authors analyzed data obtained from five double-blind, placebo-controlled studies of the efficacy and tolerability of oral sildenafil taken as required (but not more than once daily) over a 12-week to 6-month period. Two subgroups were evaluated: (a) elderly patients with ED of broad-spectrum etiology ($n=411$) and (b) elderly patients with ED and diabetes ($n=71$). Efficacy was assessed using a global efficacy question, questions 3 and 4 of the International Index of Erectile Function (IIEF) and the five sexual function domains of the IIEF. All efficacy assessments indicated that sildenafil significantly improved erectile function both in elderly patients with ED of broad-spectrum etiology and in elderly patients with ED and diabetes. The most common adverse events were mild-to-moderate headache, flushing, and dyspepsia. The rates of discontinuation due to adverse events were low and were comparable to the rates with placebo.

Beyond these oral agents, nonpharmacologic entities for treatment include intra-cavernosal injections; intraurethral suppositories, penile implants, and vacuum erection pump devices (Table 11.11, [61]). A more invasive surgical option is penile arterial bypass surgery, which has been shown to have long-term success and high overall satisfaction rates in very select patients [61]. However, all invasive treatment options can be limited by patient age, dexterity (Is he dexterous enough to perform intracavernosal injections?), fear of injections/surgery, lack of spontaneity, risk for penile injuries, priapism and fibrosis, and pain [101]. For the optimal treatment plan, it usually takes a combination of lifestyle changes, psychosocial counseling, sexual techniques, good patient–physician communication, and appropriate treatment modality.

Penile injections work well in older men. 300 men, 63–85 years of age (mean 67.1) with erectile dysfunction of organic origin were treated with penile injections [101]. Among the patients, 180 underwent first trial with injection of prostaglandin E1 (PE). Further on these 180 patients and another 120 (in total 300 patients) were treated with a triple combination of papaverine hydrochlorate, phentolamine messylate, and prostaglandin E1 (PPR). The number of responders to the injection of either PE alone or the drug combination was recorded. These authors observed a statistically significant association between the results obtained after the injection of PPR as compared to PE (χ^2 with 2 d.f.: 34.666; $P = <0.001$). A functional erection was obtained in 224/300 (74.7%) after the injection of PPR as compared to 87/180 men (48.3%) treated with PE. The average volume of PPR necessary to obtain a functional erection was 0.35+/−0.14 mL whereas that of PE was 1.3+/−0.3 mL. Thus, it appears that both the PE and PPR yielded functional erections in a significant number of older men with ED.

With respect to the implantation of penile prosthesis in older men, data suggest that this is a viable option. 174 patients received, for the first time, a penile prosthesis between 1990 and 2007 were studied [102]. Among these, 35 patients were aged > or = 70 years at prosthesis implantation. Of these, 18 patients were still alive at the time of follow-up. Using a telephone survey, patients were asked to answer the Erectile Dysfunction Inventory of Treatment Satisfaction (EDITS) as well as the International Index of Erectile Dysfunction (IIEF). In all, 15 of 18 patients were either very or somewhat satisfied (83%). At follow-up 11 out of 15 (73%) patients were using their prosthesis regularly. The mean IIEF and EDITS scores were 21.80 and 75.20, respectively. Thus, it appears in this small study, that a penile prosthesis is a viable option for the older male.

Effects of treating male ED on the partner/relationship. Data has emerged that the treatment of male ED has led to varying degrees of improved partner satisfaction as well. One hundred heterosexual couples in stable relationships, with male partners having ED based on the erectile function subscale of the International Index of Erectile Function, were randomly assigned to receive sildenafil or tadalafil for a 12-week phase, followed by another 12-week period using the alternate drug [103].

Table 11.11 Treatment options for men with erectile dysfunction (from [61])

Treatment	Cost	Advantages	Disadvantages	Recommendation
Psychosexual therapy	$50–$150/session	Noninvasive; Partner involved; Curative	Time-consuming; Patient resistance	First-line treatment; May be combined with other treatments
Oral sildenafil	$10/dose	Oral dosage; Effective	Cardiovascular disease a contraindication in some men; 1-h wait	First-line treatment; Contraindicated with nitrates
Transurethral alprostadil	$25/dose	Local therapy; Few systemic side effects	Moderately effective (43–60% with Actis[a]); Requires office training; Causes penile pain	Second-line treatment
Intracavernous alprostadil or drug mixtures[b]	$5–$25/dose	Highly effective (up to 90%); Few systemic side effects	Requires injection; High dropout rate; Can cause priapism or fibrosis; Causes penile pain	Second-line treatment
Vacuum constriction device	$150–$450/device	Least expensive; No systemic side effects	Unnatural erection; Causes petechiae; Causes numbness (20%); Trapped ejaculation	Second-line treatment
Surgical treatment				
Prosthesis (all types)	$8,000–$15,000	Highly effective	Unnatural erection (semirigid device); Infection; Requires replacement in 5–10 years; Requires anesthesia and surgery	For men not satisfied with medical treatment
Vascular surgery	$10,000–$15,000	Curative	Poor results in older men with generalized disease; Requires anesthesia and surgery	For young men with congenital or traumatic erectile dysfunction

[a]Actis is an adjustable penile-constriction device
[b]Drug mixtures contain two or three of the following drugs: papaverine, phentolamine, and alprostadil

Table 11.12 The efficacy and safety of tadalafil dosed once a day for the treatment of erectile dysfunction (adapted from [106])

	Placebo	Tadalafil 2.5 mg	Tadalafil 5 mg
Number of patients randomly assigned (N)	94	96	97
Age (years), mean (range)	58.8 (29.5–79.9)	59.8 (26.3–82.3)	60.0 (25.5–81.9)
Age >65 (n(%))	29 (31)	38 (40)	32 (33)

Male and female participants completed sexual event diaries during both study phases, and the female participants were interviewed at baseline, midpoint, and end of study. Primary outcome data were the women's final interviews during which they were asked which drug they preferred and their reasons for that preference. A total of 79.2% of the women preferred their partners' use of tadalafil, while 15.6% preferred sildenafil. Preference was not affected by age or treatment order randomization. Women preferring tadalafil reported feeling more relaxed, experiencing less pressure, and enjoying a more natural or spontaneous sexual experience as reasons for their choice. Mean number of tablets used, events recorded, events per week, and days between events were not significantly different during each study phase.

Other data corroborate these findings. A retrospective analysis [104] included data pooled from two multicenter, randomized, double-blind, placebo-controlled trials that included 505 couples (tadalafil, $n=373$; placebo, $n=132$) in which the men received tadalafil 5 mg once daily (this dosing regimen discussed a bit later) or placebo for 12 weeks. Individual Sexual Encounter Profile (SEP) diaries were completed independently by the male subject and his female partner after each sexual intercourse attempt. The mean per-subject/per-partner percentage of "yes" responses to SEP diary questions were assessed, as was agreement between subjects' and partners' responses. Subjects and partners in the tadalafil-treated group reported significantly greater improvements in the man's ability to achieve some erection, vaginal penetration, and overall sexual satisfaction compared with the placebo-treated group ($P<0.001$). For all intercourse attempts, the mean per-couple percentage of agreement for those in the tadalafil and placebo groups, respectively, was high for erection achievement (99.0% and 96.6%), vaginal penetration (98.6% and 97.4%), and overall satisfaction (84.3% and 82.8%). These authors concluded that tadalafil 5 mg taken once daily as treatment for ED improved overall satisfaction for men and their female partners. This analysis demonstrates the high concordance among couples in their responses to the man's treatment for ED.

Daily oral PDE5-I therapy for male ED: Historically, oral PDE5-I were taken on an as-needed (prn) basis. This meant that the man would take the oral PDE5-I in proximity to the anticipated sexual encounter. Data emerged recently that confirmed that oral, daily tadalafil, both 2.5 and 5 mg, improved erectile function and might be a reasonable alternative to prn dosing [104–106]. While no specific studies have been performed in aging men, older men were included in clinical trial that examined daily dosing (Table 11.12, adapted from [105]) and appeared to receive benefit from daily tadalafil. As is seen in this dataset, the efficacy and safety of tadalafil, dosed once a day for the treatment of erectile dysfunction, was assessed in a randomized, double-blind, placebo-controlled, parallel-design study at 15 US centers. Following a 4-week treatment-free run-in period, patients (18 years of age) were randomly assigned to 24 weeks treatment with tadalafil 2.5 mg, tadalafil 5 mg, or placebo. Primary efficacy endpoints were changed at 24 weeks in International Index of Erectile Function Erectile Function (EF) Domain score and mean per-patient percentage "yes" responses to Sexual Encounter Profile diary questions 2 and 3. Tadalafil significantly improved erectile function compared with placebo for all three co-primary efficacy endpoints. Few patients discontinued because of adverse events (2.1%, placebo; 6.3%, tadalafil 2.5 mg; 4.1%, tadalafil 5 mg). Common treatment-emergent adverse events (5%) were nasopharyngitis, influenza, viral gastro-enteritis, and back pain. Tadalafil 2.5 and 5 mg, dosed once a day for 24 weeks, was well tolerated and significantly improved erectile function.

Daily dosing with tadalafil has changed the ED treatment paradigm. Evidence for improvement in various outcome measures as seen in the following study [106]. An efficacy study of tadalafil (5 mg once daily) for treating erectile dysfunction included sexual satisfaction and psychosocial outcome measures such as Treatment satisfaction (THX) domain of Sexual Life Quality Questionnaire, Self-Esteem And Relationship (SEAR) questionnaire, Sexual Encounter Profile questions 4 (SEP4; hardness satis-faction) and 5 (SEP5; overall satisfaction), intercourse satisfaction (IS) and overall satisfaction (OS) domains of International Index of Erectile Function (IIEF), and part-ner SEP question 3 (pSEP3). After a 4-week run-in phase, participants were random-ized to receive either tadalafil ($N = 264$) or placebo ($N = 78$) for 12 weeks. Participants and partners were more satisfied (THX) with tadalafil (75 and 73, respectively) than with placebo (51 and 55, respectively, $P < 0.001$). Statistically significant improve-ments in sexual relationship, confidence, self-esteem and overall relationship (SEAR), in addition to IS, OS, SEP5, and pSEP3 for tadalafil compared with placebo ($P < 0.001$) correlated with erectile function (EF) improvement (assessed by change from baseline in IIEF-EF score). Tadalafil significantly improved treatment and sexual satisfaction, while improving multiple outcomes measured by SEAR. Daily tadalafil for the treat-ment of male ED was FDA approved in 2008 (http://newsroom.lilly.com/releasede-tail.cfm?releaseid=285378) and is a viable option for the treatment of male ED.

New concept: daily tadalafil for both ED and BPH/ LUTS. As men age, the pros-tate enlarges and produces a variety of symptoms termed LUTS. LUTS is character-ized by urinary frequency, urgency, weak stream, and nocturia [107]. LUTS is prevalent in more than half of men over the age of 50 years. BPH and LUTS significantly decrease quality of life in aging men and may worsen to acute urinary retention requiring emergency care. Treatment of LUTS has centered on oral alpha blockers as first-line therapy to reduce the LUTS [108]. Alpha blockers include such drugs as doxazosin, terazosin, tamsulosin, alfuzosin, and silodosin [108]. Interestingly, epidemiologic studies indicate a strong association between LUTS and male sexual dysfunction (ED and ejaculatory dysfunction) suggesting a com-mon pathophysiologic theme [109, 110]. In addition, both erectile and ejaculatory disorders appear more frequently in men in conjunction with symptoms of moderate to severe LUTS [109, 110]. Although the exact mechanisms in regard to how LUTS

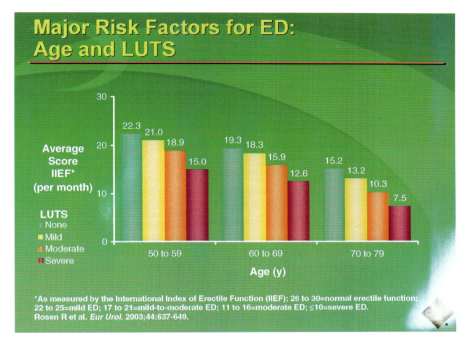

Fig. 11.6 Data shows average score for Erectile Function (as measured by IIEF) in each age group amongst men without LUTS (*left column*). As expected, a clear decline in Erectile Function with increasing age is observed. Within each age group, the average score for Erectile Function (IIEF) decreases significantly with increasing severity of LUTS. The same relationship hold true for ejaculatory dysfunction (courtesy of testosteroneupdate.org.)

affect sexual function are not clear, there appears to be a direct relationship between the two. This is especially evident when sexual problems are encountered or exacerbated by management of LUTS, (Fig 11.6, [110]). The Multinational Survey of the Aging Male (MSAM-7) was conducted in the United States and 6 European countries to systematically investigate the relationship between LUTS and sexual dysfunction in older men aged 50–80 years [110]. LUTS and sexual function were assessed using validated symptom scales, including the International Prostate Symptom Score (IPSS) for LUTS, and the Danish Prostatic Symptom Score and the IIEF for sexual function. A total of 12,815 surveys were included in the analysis. The men's self-ratings of erectile function were stratified according to the severity of LUTS. An IIEF total score of 26–30 indicates normal erectile function, and a score of 10 or less indicates severe ED. As expected, there was a gradual worsening of erectile function with increased age. However, within each age group, there was a clear, statistically important relationship between the severity of LUTS and erectile capacity. As LUTS worsened, so did erectile function. Moreover, the relationship between sexual problems and LUTS was independent of comorbidities such as diabetes, hypertension, cardiac disease, and hypercholesterolemia [110].

There was a clear age-related decline in male sexual function, both erectile function and ejaculatory function, seen with aging. The decline in sexual function with aging was exacerbated by worsening LUTS. For example, (Fig. 11.6), if a man in the age bracket 50–59 has no LUTS, his erectile function score was quite good at 22.3. As the LUTS take effect, the worsening of the LUTS symptoms now demonstrated that the same man has a worsening of his erectile function. Indeed, with moderate LUTS, the erection score drops to 18.9, a 15% decline in erectile function (Fig. 11.6). The clinical implications of these recent studies suggest that a man who presents with LUTS should be carefully evaluated for the presence of sexual problems and vice versa.

The possible pathophysiologic mechanistic relationship between LUTS and ED is the subject of intense investigation [111]. One plausible common mechanism is that both organs (the prostate and the penis) contain PDE5, and either upregulation of the intrinsic PDE5 enzyme or loss of intrinsic PDE5-I protein may cause exacerbation of prostate smooth contraction and penile corpus cavernosum contraction. Excessive contraction prevents the relaxation needed for penile erection and the prostate relaxation needed for the patient to void. The PDE5 and PDE5-I mechanisms are well elucidated for the penile corpus cavernosum smooth muscle [61], but are not as clearly defined in the prostate. cGMP and PDE5 have recently been identified via immunohistochemistry, mRNA, and Western blot in the rat and human prostate [111–115] PDE5 inhibitors have been shown to relax prostate tissue in vitro [111–115].

Uckert et al. [112] performed the following experiments. Using the organ bath technique, the effects of increasing concentrations (1 nM to 10 μM) of the PDE5 inhibitors sildenafil, tadalafil, and vardenafil and the PDE4 inhibitors rolipram and RP 73401 on the tension induced by norepinephrine (NE, 40 μM) of prostate strip preparations were investigated. The accumulation of cyclic guanosine monophosphate and cyclic adenosine monophosphate in response to drug exposure was determined by radioimmunoassays, The tension induced by NE was dose dependently reversed by the drugs with the following rank order of efficacy: tadalafil greater than RP 73401greater than rolipram greater than or equal to vardenafil greater than sildenafil. The maximal reversion of tension values ranged from 52.3% (tadalafil) to 17% (sildenafil). Of the PDE inhibitors, only tadalafil induced a 50% reversion of the initial tension. The most prominent enhancement in tissue cyclic adenosine monophosphate was registered in response to RP 73401 (11-fold), and cyclic guanosine monophosphate levels were significantly elevated by tadalafil, vardenafil, and sildenafil (28-fold, 12-fold, and threefold, respectively) [112].

Zhang et al. [114] investigated the effect of testoserone (T) on smooth muscle (SM) contractile and regulatory signaling pathways including PDE5 expression and functional activity in prostate in male rats (sham-operated, surgically- castrated and castrated with T supplementation). In vitro organ bath studies, real-time RT-PCR, Western blot analysis, and immunohistochemistry were performed. PDE5 was immunolocalized exclusively in the prostate stroma (Fig. 11.7). The PDE5-I zaprinast significantly increased prostate strip relaxation to the nitric oxide donor sodium nitroprusside (SNP) in control but not castrated rats. But SNP alone was more effective on castrated rats, comparable with sham treated with SNP plus zaprinast. T supplementation prevented or restored all above changes, including

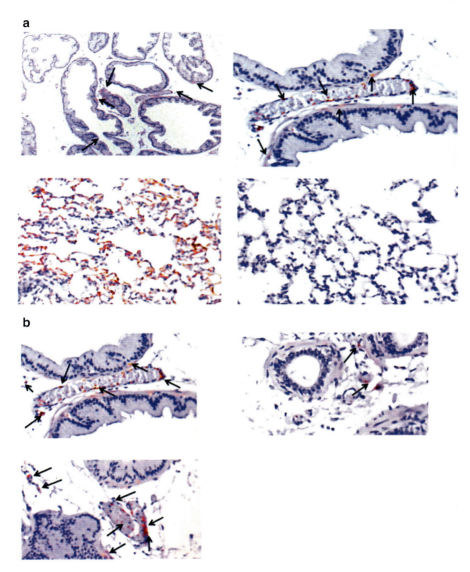

Fig. 11.7 Immunolocalization of phosphodiesterase 5 (PDE5) in rat ventral prostate. (**a**) *top*: PDE5 positive immunoreactivity in the prostatic stroma from sham-operated rats with magnification × 100 (*left*) and × 400 (*right*). (**a**) *bottom left*: positive PDE5 control (rat lung, magnification × 400); (**a**) *bottom right*: negative IgG control staining (rat lung, magnification × 400). B: PDE5 immunopositivity in the prostatic stroma from sham (*top left*), castrated (*top right*), and castrated + T (*bottom left*) rats with magnification × 400 (from Zhang et al. [114])

SNP and   prinast in vitro responsiveness. These data show that T positively regulates PD   xpression and functional activities in prostate, and T ablation not only
suppress   ostate size but also reduces prostatic SM contractility, with several
potenti   contraction/relaxation pathways implicated. Zaprinast findings

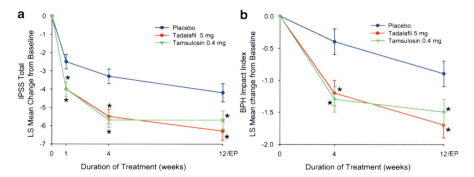

Fig. 11.8 Changes from baseline in (**a**) total International Prostate Symptom Score and (**b**) Benign Prostatic Hyperplasia Impact Index. Data represent the least squares mean change plus or minus standard error. *LS* least squares; *EP* end point; *ANCOVA* analysis of covariance.*$p < 0.05$ vs. placebo based on ANCOVA (from Oelke et al. [117])

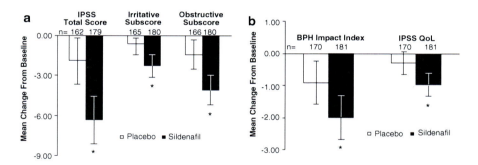

Fig. 11.9 Change in LUTS scores from baseline to end of treatment. Patients completed I-PSS irritative and obstructive subscales (**a**), and BPHII and I-PSS QOL question (**b**) at baseline and after 12 weeks of randomized treatment. Maximum I-PSS score is 35 points, maximum irritative subscore is 15 points, and maximum obstructive subscore is 20 points. Maximum BPHII score is 13 points. I-PSS QOL question asks "If you were to spend the rest of your life with your urinary condition just the way it is now, how would you feel about that?" and it is scored on 0 to 6-point scale. Lower I-PSS and BPHII scores indicate fewer LUTS, less bother, and better QOL. Greater decreases in LS mean scores on each set of questions indicate better treatment outcome. Data are shown as LS mean change with 95% CI. *Asterisk* indicates sildenafil change in LS mean score vs. placebo change in score $p < 0.0001$ (from McVary et al. [120])

strongly suggest a major role for PDE5/cGMP in this signaling cascade. These data support PDE5 inhibition as a potential mechanism for the treatment of BPH.

There are data now that suggest clinical LUTS may benefit from ED treatment with PDE5 inhibition. Tadalafil was recently approved by the FDA for daily use for the treatment of both BPH/LUTS and ED [116]. Data suggest [117, 118] that tadalafil can improve LUTS in a similar manner to alpha blockers (Fig. 11.8), without the alpha blocker side effects (though there are the PDE5-I side effects). Tadalafil does not change the PSA at a 1-year time point [119]. Sildenafil (Fig 11.9, [120]) and vardenafil also improve BPH/ LUTS symptoms but have not yet cleared the FDA regulatory hurdles for the BPH indication [120, 121].

The tadalafil vs the alpha blocker tamsulosin data are as follows [117]. A randomized, double-blind, international, placebo-controlled, parallel-group study assessed men ≥45 years of age with LUTS/BPH, IPSS ≥13, and maximum urinary flow rate (Q(max)) ≥4 to ≤15 mL/s. Following screening and washout, if needed, subjects completed a 4-weeks placebo run-in before randomization to placebo ($n = 172$), tadalafil 5 mg ($n = 171$), or tamsulosin 0.4 mg ($n = 168$) once daily for 12 weeks.

IPSS significantly improved versus placebo through 12 weeks with tadalafil (-2.1; $p = 0.001$; primary efficacy outcome) and tamsulosin (-1.5; $p = 0.023$) and as early as 1 week (tadalafil and tamsulosin both -1.5; $p < 0.01$). BPH Impact Index significantly improved versus placebo at first assessment (week 4) with tadalafil (-0.8; $p < 0.001$) and tamsulosin (-0.9; $p < 0.001$) and through 12 weeks (tadalafil -0.8, $p = 0.003$; tamsulosin -0.6, $p = 0.026$) (Fig 11.6). The IPSS Quality-of-Life Index and the Treatment Satisfaction Scale-BPH improved significantly vs. placebo with tadalafil (both $p < 0.05$) but not with tamsulosin (both $p > 0.1$). The International Index of Erectile Function-Erectile Function domain improved versus placebo with tadalafil (4.0; $p < 0.001$) but not tamsulosin (-0.4; $p = 0.699$). Q(max) increased significantly versus placebo with both tadalafil (2.4 mL/s; $p = 0.009$) and tamsulosin (2.2 mL/s; $p = 0.014$). Adverse event profiles were consistent with previous reports. This study was limited in not being powered to directly compare tadalafil vs. tamsulosin. The data suggest that monotherapy with tadalafil or tamsulosin resulted in significant and numerically similar improvements vs. placebo in LUTS/BPH and Q(max). However, only tadalafil improved erectile dysfunction. Thus, daily PDE5-I therapy with tadalafil is a viable option for the treatment of both ED and BPH/LUTS.

Treatment of Hypogonadism: Treatment of the Aging Male with Testosterone

Treatment for men with symptomatic hypogonadism is testosterone supplementation. There are multiple methods of delivery including injectable, implantable pellets, buccal, transdermal patches, and gels [122]. Although side effects exist, testosterone replacement therapy has been shown to improve muscle mass, energy levels, and bone strength. In older men with significant hypogonadism, testosterone treatment has been effective in enhancing the strength and maintenance of erections [123–127]. In the absence of hypogonadism, testosterone supplementation has been shown to improve the response to sildenafil [125, 126]. Aversa et al. demonstrated that in patients with ED and low-normal androgen levels, short-term testosterone administration increased testosterone (total and fr   levels and improved the erectile response to sildenafil likely by increasing   ial inflow to the penis during stimulation [128]. Furthermore, one review   d that transdermal therapy appears to be more effective than intramuscular   ery methods [129].

As noted above, controversy exists regarding the lower end of normal for hypogonadism along with the normal levels for the aging male. Seftel et al attempted to provide guidance regarding the therapeutic targets for T replacement ([130], Fig. 11.10). Hypogonadal male subjects from the Testim phase 3 studies (total T < or = 300 ng/dL, $n = 406$, mean age 58 years) reporting one or more symptoms of low testosterone were randomized to T gel (50 mg/day and 100 mg/day), T patch, or placebo. Twenty-four-hour pharmacokinetic profiles for T were obtained. The three primary end points evaluated at 30 and 90 days posttreatment included a significant change in the frequency of intercourse and nighttime erections per 7-day week as well as a change in sexual desire measured on a Likert-type scale and calculated as a mean daily score. At day 30, a significant increase from baseline in sexual desire was noted for those on 100 mg/day T gel compared with those on 50 mg/day T gel, T patch, or placebo (1.2 vs. 0.4, 0.7, and 0.4, respectively). A significant increase from baseline in the frequency of nighttime erections was also noted for those on 100 mg/day T gel compared with those on 50 mg/day T gel or placebo (51% of subjects in the 100 mg/day T gel group had an increase in frequency vs. 30% for the 50 mg/day T gel group and 26% in the placebo group). Finally, a significant increase from baseline in the frequency of intercourse was evidenced for those on 100 mg/day T gel compared with those on T patch or placebo (39% of subjects in the 100 mg/day T gel group had an increase in frequency vs. 21% for the T patch group and 24% in the placebo group). Similar results were seen for 100 mg/day T gel at day 90 for sexual desire and nighttime erections vs. placebo. These data demonstrate a clear relationship between restoring serum T concentrations and improvement in certain parameters of sexual function. We propose that threshold T levels are needed in order to significantly affect improvements in sexual functioning. This threshold level appeared to be approximately 400 ng/dL for nighttime erections, 500 ng/dL for sexual intercourse, and 600 ng/dL for sexual desire. In all three parameters, there was no significant difference in sexual function between the group of subjects with the lowest serum T levels (0–300 ng/dL) and the group of subjects with the next highest serum T level (300–400 ng/dL for nighttime erections, 300–500 ng/dL for sexual intercourse, and 300–600 ng/dL for sexual desire). The data are depicted in Fig. 11.10.

New formulations of T gels exist including Androgel 1.62%, Testim, Axiron, and Fortesta. Testosterone patches (Androderm) are available as along with buccal T preparations (Striant), subcutaneous pellets (Testopel), and standard intramuscular injections [131–133]. Most authorities recommend checking T levels, a CBC (or Hb/Hct) and a PSA at some designated point, along with performance of a digital rectal examination postinception of T replacement therapy [35].

There is great variability in insurance coverage for T replacement products. Further, the FDA has recently issued a "black box" warning regarding the possibility of transference of the T gel once applied by the patient to his body, to a partner or child. This can happen when the T gel is applied to an exposed skin surface and the patient comes into contact with the partner/child. The gels take about 2–6 h to dry once applied to the skin; this appropriate counseling must be provided to the patient when prescribing T replacement therapy [134].

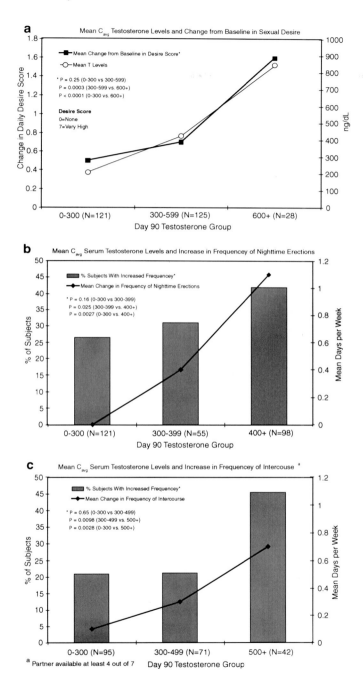

Fig. 11.10 Mean change from baseline for daily sexual desire score and mean C_{avg} (0–24 h) serum testosterone levels (ng/dL) (**a**), and percentage of subjects with increased frequency and mean change in frequency for nighttime erections (**b**) and intercourse (**c**) (from Seftel et al. [130])

In general, most of the T replacement products are well tolerated by the patient. Individual gels may have a side effect specific to its product such as skin irritation, fragrance, application site, time to full absorption, etc. The T patches may also create a bit of skin irritation, but are a reasonable option for the properly selected patient. The buccal preparation is a twice daily application to the inner gum. The T pellets are subcutaneous injections usually performed at 3–4 month intervals. The standard intramuscular injections of T are injected by either the patient or caregiver at 1–3 week intervals. The reader is encouraged to evaluate each specific product to gain familiarity with these compounds.

Treatment endpoints usually include T levels in the therapeutic range and relief of symptom (s). T levels can be raised to the higher therapeutic range if symptom relief is not accomplished with initial dosing regimens.

The most T replacement side effects include local skin reactions to the gels, patches or IM injections, polycythemia, worsening of BPH/LUTS symptoms, increases in serum PSA, pedal edema, gynecomastia, transient oligo or azoospermia, and worsening of sleep apnea.

While T replacement therapy is contraindicated in men with known prostate cancer, there is a movement afoot to offer T replacement therapy to specific men who had undergone treatment for their prostate cancer. This is an extremely controversial area that is still under investigation [135].

Recent data from the testosterone in older men "TOM" trial has created some concern regarding the beneficial effects of testosterone replacement in older, frail men [136]. These authors studied community-dwelling men, 65 years of age or older, with limitations in mobility and a total serum testosterone level of 100–350 ng/dL (3.5–12.1 nmol/L) or a free serum testosterone level of less than 50 pg/mL (173 pmol/L). These men were randomly assigned to receive placebo gel or testosterone gel, to be applied daily for 6 months. The study premise was that testosterone supplementation has been shown to increase muscle mass and strength in healthy older men. The safety and efficacy of testosterone treatment in older men who have limitations in mobility have not been studied. Adverse events were categorized with the use of the Medical Dictionary for Regulatory Activities classification.

The data and safety monitoring board recommended that the trial be discontinued early because there was a significantly higher rate of adverse cardiovascular events in the testosterone group than in the placebo group. A total of 209 men (mean age, 74 years) were enrolled at the time the trial was terminated. At baseline, there was a high prevalence of hypertension, diabetes, hyperlipidemia, and obesity among the participants. During the course of the study, the testosterone group had higher rates of cardiac, respiratory, and dermatologic events than did the placebo group. A total of 23 subjects in the testosterone group, as compared with five in the placebo group, had cardiovascular-related adverse events. The relative risk of a cardiovascular-related adverse event remained constant throughout the 6-month treatment period. As compared with the placebo group, the testosterone group had significantly greater improvements in leg-press and chest-press strength and in stair climbing while carrying a load. The authors concluded that in this population of older men with limitations in mobility and a high prevalence of chronic disease, the application of a testosterone gel was associated with an increased risk of cardiovascular adverse events. The small size of the trial and the unique population prevent broader inferences from being made about the safety of testosterone therapy.

One must weigh the data presented in the TOM trial with those data provided earlier regarding testosterone a CV symptom improvement [78, 79]. These data suggest that low T is associated with worse long-term morbidity and mortality [38] and T replacement therapy may offer some cardiovascular and cognitive benefit. T replacement therapy appears to offer some metabolic benefits in the areas of CV disease, diabetes, and the metabolic syndrome [137, 138].

Other controversial issues surround the patients with late onset hypogonadism, some authorities feed that patients with serum total testosterone levels below 8 nmol/L (230 ng/dL) will usually benefit from testosterone treatment. Total testosterone levels between 8 and 12 nmol/L (230–350 ng/dL) warrant repeat measurement of total testosterone with SHBG to calculate free testosterone or free testosterone by equilibrium dialysis. Total testosterone level above 12 nmol/(350 ng/dL) may not require substitution [84]. This is another controversial area of study.

Treatment of ejaculatory disorders: With increasing interest and clinical research in male sexual disorders, it has become clear that not only psychological but also organic, neurobiological, and genetic factors may play an important role in premature ejaculation (PE, [139]). Premature ejaculation (PE) is a very common sexual dysfunction among patients, and with varying prevalence estimates ranging from 3 to 20%. Although psychological issues are present in most patients with premature PE, as a cause or as a consequence, research on the effects of psychological approaches for PE has in general not been controlled or randomized and is lacking in long-term follow-up [140]. A recent Cochrane review has discussed psychosocial interventions for premature ejaculation [140]. The authors noted that there was weak and inconsistent evidence regarding the effectiveness of psychological interventions for the treatment of premature ejaculation. Three of the four included randomized controlled studies of psychotherapy for PE reported our primary outcome (Improvement in IELT), and the majority have a small sample size. The early success reports (97.8%) of Masters and Johnson could not be replicated. One study found a significant improvement from baseline in the duration of intercourse, sexual satisfaction, and sexual function with a new functional-sexological treatment and behavior therapy compared to waiting list. One study showed that the combination of chlorpromazine and behavioral therapy was superior to chlorpromazine alone. Randomized trials with larger group samples are still needed to further confirm or deny the current available evidence for psychological interventions for treating PE.

FDA-approved oral therapy for PE is currently not available. Dapoxetine was studied several years ago as a potential option [141]. Dapoxetine is a potent SSRI, which is administered on demand 1–3 h before planned sexual contact. Dapoxetine is rapidly absorbed and eliminated, resulting in minimal accumulation and has dose-proportional pharmacokinetics, which are unaffected by multiple dosing. Dapoxetine 30 and 60 mg has been evaluated in five randomized, double-blind, placebo-controlled studies in 6,081 men aged > or = 18 years. Outcome measures included stopwatch-measured intravaginal ejaculatory latency time (IELT), Premature Ejaculation

Profile (PEP) items, clinical global impression of change (CGIC) in PE, and adverse events. Mean IELT, all PEP items and CGIC improved significantly with both doses of dapoxetine vs. placebo ($p<0.001$ for all). The most common adverse events included nausea, dizziness, and headache, and evaluation of validated rated scales demonstrated no SSRI class-related effects with dapoxetine use [134]. Dapoxetine did not receive FDA approval for use in the USA but has received approval in several other countries. (http://www.dapoxetinereview.com/dapoxetine_fda.html)

STDs in Aging Populations

Sexually transmitted disease (STDs) has become more prevalent as people get older and reengage in sexual activity. The Centers for Disease Control and Prevention (CDC) report that the number of cases of acquired immunodeficiency syndrome (AIDS) has risen from 739 cases in 1999 to 846 in 2009 for adults aged 65 years and older [142]. Although HIV/AIDS transmission through blood transfusions has decreased, other sources of cases by sexual intercourse and multiple sexual partners have increased the number of documented cases [143]. Risk factors for HIV/AIDS in the aging population are the same as those for younger adults—sexual contact, multiple partners, STDs, substance abuse, and intravenous drug use.

Older people are especially prone to the sequelae of HIV/AIDS largely because of the decline of humoral and cell-mediated defense mechanisms associated with the aging process [12, 13]. The geriatric population is more susceptible to opportunistic infections such as mycobacterium tuberculosis, herpes zoster, and cytomegalovirus. Postmenopausal women are especially at risk for contracting HIV during sexual intercourse because of decreased lubrication and vaginal wall thinning [144–146]. There is a more aggressive pattern of progression after HIV seroconversion with a lesser response to antiretroviral treatment agents. There are also additional comorbidities that the elderly have predisposes them to an early and rapid demise once afflicted with AIDS as multiple systems are compromised quicker. In fact many elderly die of AIDS before a diagnosis of HIV infection is even made [144–146].

Treatment of HIV/AIDS in elderly patients is the same as in the general population. There is a greater propensity for interactions and adverse reactions because older people are usually taking additional medications for their comorbidities. In older adults, antiretroviral therapies should be started at low dosage and increased gradually under close monitoring. Unfortunately, this patient population has the burden of combined compromised health and compromised cognitive ability to sometimes adequately deal with the initial diagnosis of HIV and also the physical and emotional stress of going through the treatment plan [6]. They require additional support and more importantly, a discussion weighing the risks and benefits of HIV/AIDS treatment in the context of end-of-life issues.

Because of the significant risks of HIV and other STDs in the geriatric population, it should be stressed to older adults that age in and of itself is not a barrier against these diseases. In the older patient who experiences memory loss, a workup for syphilis should be conducted in additional to evaluating for other neurologic conditions [144, 145]. Other more common STDs, such as gonococcal urethritis, vaginitis, trichomoniasis, and chlamydia, are as ubiquitous amongst the geriatric population as its younger counterpart and should be appropriately treated when found [5]. In nursing homes and assisted living facilities, sexual assault of the cognitively impaired individual should be considered if he or she develops STDs [144, 145]. These various issues and statistics underscore the importance of affirming safe sexual practices amongst the geriatric population by the general practitioner.

Comorbidities

Comorbid disease processes can have a significant negative impact on sexual health, especially in the geriatric population. Disease states usually cause low energy levels, fatigue, pain, impairment, muscle weakness, and psychologic disturbances that hamper a sexual relationship [146, 147]. Conditions requiring surgical intervention can affect anatomic functions (e.g., amputations, colostomy, urostomy, etc.) and distort self-image (e.g., scars, burns) and lower self-esteem, causing problems with sexual attraction [11]. Often times, patients are prohibited from significant sexual contact after the resolution of a disease state. Examples include the post-prostatectomy patient as the patient may be unable to get an erection or the post-myocardial infarction (MI) patient because he or she is fearful of getting a second MI during intercourse. Updated guidelines for the clinician have recently been published to assist with the post-MI patient and other patients afflicted with CV disease who wish to resume sexual activity [54–57]. A cardiovascular evaluation may be required to assess the patients' physical capability and endurance requirements necessary to resume sexual intercourse. Both sexual partners should be cognizant and comfortable with sexual activities after one partner undergoes a life altering condition or surgery.

Post-CVA patients may have paralysis or reduced libido and diminished orgasms. Post-stroke weakness can be unilateral and can sometimes be addressed by alternative positioning while engaging in sexual activities [146, 147]. Concerns also exist that medications used to treat certain conditions may result in sexual dysfunction.

Diabetes, a significant contributing factor for ED in men, can also negatively impact women's sexuality. DM can cause a decrease of vaginal secretions and reduce libido. Different sequelae of DM such as retinopathy leading to blindness, amputations, renal failure requiring dialysis, peripheral neuropathy, and chronic pain can also hamper sexual functioning [12]. Chronic arthritis can cause pain and joint swelling, limiting range of motion during sex [11].

Postsurgical patients, including all forms of surgery, may experience side effects such as pain, scarring, and lymphedema, all of which can interfere with a patient's interest and ability to engage in sexual activities. The patient's partner may also find it difficult to cope with his or her partner's sexual difficulties and inadequacies and may not feel any sexual attraction under those circumstances [146, 147]. There is a heavy toll on both the physical and emotional components of postsurgical relationship. Most post-hysterectomy women found less desire and enjoyment during intercourse after their surgeries; however, a minority had improved sexual activity because their pre-hysterectomy symptoms and pain were gone [148].

In men, the most common noncutaneous malignancy is prostate cancer. With any of the treatment modalities offered, including open or robotic radical prostatectomy, external beam radiation, or brachytherapy, there is significant concern for incontinence, impotence, and diminished libido [149]. Prostatectomy, if not nerve-sparing, may inhibit return of spontaneous erections. In addition, some men consider prostatectomy as an assault on his male sexuality and suffer considerable psychological detriment postoperatively, thereby diminishing sexual desire and function [150]. Urinary incontinence, as a result of radical prostatectomy, can also impact sexual behavior negatively in the elderly. Nocturia, bedwetting, and fear of incontinence during sex can all decrease sexual desire and activity. The use of Kegel exercises to improve continence and appropriate medications can sometimes overcome these side effects and may lead to improvement in sexual function in the older man [151]. The post-prostatectomy male has the same options for the treatment of erectile dysfunction listed above for the elderly patient.

In addition to organic comorbidities, one must consider chronic psychologic disease as associated with sexual dysfunction. Depression and anxiety are serious and prevalent disorders in American men and women [152]. Like the story of the chicken and the egg, depression and anxiety can precede and cause sexual dysfunction as well as be a result of sexual dysfunction. Although psychotherapy and pharmacotherapy can provide substantial relief and clinical improvement in disease extent, some antidepressants have sexual side effects, making these drugs counterproductive in treating sexual dysfunction.

Religious and Cultural Aspects

In the aging population, many of the tenets and religious philosophies taught to them in childhood play a significant role in their adulthood. Some cultures paint sexuality and its expression as a picture of sin and darkness on a religious basis. Others allow for more freedom and insight. In some settings, prior religious teachings can detract the elderly from experiencing a satisfactory sexual relationship because of feelings of guilt and repression. It is therefore important for urologists and physicians to address these religious feelings and attempt to incorporate the treatment of sexual dysfunction in a manner that is understandable and complementary to the patient's religious background [26].

Conclusions and Future Research

In summary, sexuality still plays a predominant role in the health and general well-being of the older adult. There are a multitude of physical, psychological, emotional, and spiritual implications of a healthy sex life as men and women age [153]. A healthy sense of sexuality in the aging adult provides a more fulfilled lifestyle and significantly improves quality of life. Although there are challenges and diseases that can affect sexuality as one age, those obstacles can be treated and sometimes overcome outright. As more and more Americans live longer, it becomes increasingly more important that the urologist and general physician come to terms with the fact that sex life does not disappear with old age and that many elderly people have and enjoy a satisfactory sexual experience. With a balanced and healthy lifestyle combined with new advances in medicine, sexual wellbeing can play a crucial role in advanced age.

Finally, the outcome measures used by the FDA for the FSD drug development process remain a significant challenge in the field of FSD. A recent review highlights some of the issues [154]. Assessing the sexual response in women with FSDs in clinical trials remains difficult. Part of the challenge is the development of meaningful and valid end points that capture the complexity of women's sexual response. The authors wished to highlight the shortcomings of daily diaries and the limitations of satisfying sexual events (SSEs) as primary end points in clinical trials of women with HSDD as recommended by the Food and Drug Administration (FDA) in their draft guidance on standards for clinical trials in women with FSD. Nine placebo-controlled randomized trials in women with HSDD were reviewed: seven with transdermal testosterone and two with flibanserin. In four trials, all using transdermal testosterone 300 µg/day had agreement between changes in SSEs, desire, and distress. In five studies (testosterone 300 µg/day, $n=2$; testosterone 150 µg/day, $n=1$; flibanserin $n=2$), changes in SSEs did not correlate with changes in desire and/or distress and vice versa. It should be noted that in the flibanserin trials, SSEs did correlate with desire assessed using the FSFI but not when it was assessed using the eDiary. The authors concluded that the findings in the literature do not uniformly support the recommendations from the FDA draft guidance to use diary measures in clinical trials of HSDD as primary endpoints. Patient-reported outcomes appear to be better suited to capture the multidimensional and more subjective information collected in trials of FSD [153]. Future research will hopefully answer these study endpoint and other research questions.

Epilogue

The authors are indebted to the numerous researchers who have contributed to this field. This chapter reflects their significant time commitment to the field of sexual medicine.

The keys to success in this discipline are to remember that these patients form a distinct group that requires understanding and patience to help them achieve their goals.

References

1. Fowles DG, Greenberg S. A profile of older Americans: 2010. Administration on Aging, Department of Health and Human Services, 2010.
2. Lindau ST, Laumann EO, Levinson W, Waite LJ. Synthesis of scientific disciplines in pursuit of health: the Interactive Biopsychosocial Model. Perspect Biol Med. 2003;46 Suppl 3:S74–86.
3. Laumann EO, Paik A, Rosen RC. Sexual dysfunction in the United States: prevalence and predictors. JAMA. 1999;281(6):537–44.
4. Lindau ST, Schumm P, Laumann EO, Levinson W, O'Muircheartaigh CA, Waite LJ. A study of sexuality and health among older adults in the United States. N Engl J Med. 2007;357(8): 762–74.
5. Rienzo B. The impact of aging on human sexuality. J Sch Health. 1985;55(2):66–8.
6. Lenahan P, Ellwood A. Sexual health and aging. Clin Fam Pract. 2004;6(4):917–39.
7. Laumann EO, Paik A, Glasser DB, Kang JH, Wang T, Levinson B, et al. A cross-national study of subjective sexual well-being among older women and men: findings from the Global Study of Sexual Attitudes and Behaviors. Arch Sex Behav. 2006;35(2):145–61.
8. Nusbaum MRH, Gamble GR, Pathman DE. Seeking medical help for sexual concerns: frequency, barriers, and missed opportunities. J Fam Pract. 2002;51:706.
9. Lindau ST, Leitsch SA, Lundberg KL, Jerome J. Older women's attitudes, behavior, and communication about sex and HIV: a community-based study. J Womens Health (Larchmt). 2006;15(6):747–53.
10. Gott M, Hinchliff S, Galena E. General practitioner attitudes to discussing sexual health issues with older people. Soc Sci Med. 2004;58(11):2093–103.
11. Kaiser F. Sexuality practice of geriatrics. 3rd ed. Philadelphia: WB Saunders; 1998. p. 48–56.
12. Ginsberg TB. Aging and sexuality. Med Clin North Am. 2006;90(5):1025–36.
13. Drench M, Losee R. Sexuality and sexual capacities of elderly people. Rehabil Nurs. 1996; 21(3):118–23.
14. Jung A, Schill WB. Male sexuality with advancing age. Eur J Obstet Gynecol Reprod Biol. 2004;113:123–5.
15. Mulligan T, Reddy S, Gulur PV, Godschalk M. Disorders of male sexual function. Clin Geriatr Med. 2003;19(3):473–81.
16. Masters W, Johnson V. Sex and the aging process. J Am Geriatr Soc. 1981;29:385–90.
17. Pariser S, Niedermier J. Sex and the mature woman. J Womens Health. 1998;7(7):849–59.
18. Wilson MM. Menopause. Clin Geriatr Med. 2003;19(3):483–506.
19. West SL, D'Aloisio AA, Agans RP, Kalsbeek WD, Borisov NN, Thorp JM. Prevalence of low sexual desire and hypoactive sexual desire disorder in a nationally representative sample of US women. Arch Intern Med. 2008;168(13):1441–9.
20. Trompeter SE, Bettencourt R, Barrett-Connor E. Sexual activity and satisfaction in healthy community-dwelling older women. Am J Med. 2012;125(1):37–43.e1.
21. Noblett KI, Ostergard DR. Gynecologic disorders. In: Hazzard W, Blass J, Ettinger Jr W, Halter J, Ouslander J, editors. Principles of geriatric medicine and gerontology. 4th ed. New York: McGraw-Hill; 1999. p. 797–807.
22. Robinson JG, Wallace R, Limacher M, Ren H, Cochrane B, Wassertheil-Smoller S, et al. Cardiovascular risk in women with non-specific chest pain (from the Women's Health Initiative Hormone Trials). Am J Cardiol. 2008;102(6):693–9.
23. Bernstein L. The risk of breast, endometrial and ovarian cancer in users of hormonal preparations. Basic Clin Pharmacol Toxicol. 2006;98(3):288–96.
24. Johannes CB, McKinlay JB, et al. Incidence of erectile dysfunction in men 40 to 69 years old: longitudinal results from the Massachusetts Male Aging Study. J Urol. 2000;163:460–3.
25. McKinlay JB, et al. The worldwide prevalence and epidemiology of erectile dysfunction. Int J Impot Res. 2000;12 Suppl 4:S6.
26. Hogan R. Influences of culture on sexuality. Nurs Clin North Am. 1982;17(3):365–76.
27. Laumann EO, et al. The social organization of sexuality: sexual practices in the United States. Chicago: University of Chicago Press; 1994. p. 370.

28. Feldman HA, et al. Impotence and its medical and psychosocial correlates: results of the Massachusetts Male Aging study. J Urol. 1994;151:54.
29. Waldinger MD. Recent advances in the classification, neurobiology and treatment of premature ejaculation. Adv Psychosom Med. 2008;29:50–69.
30. Waldinger MD, McIntosh J, Schweitzer DH. A five-nation survey to assess the distribution of the intravaginal ejaculatory latency time among the general male population. J Sex Med. 2009;6(10):2888–95.
31. Althof SE, Abdo CH, Dean J, Hackett G, McCabe M, McMahon CG et al. International Society for Sexual Medicine's guidelines for the diagnosis and treatment of premature ejaculation. J Sex Med. 2010;7(9):2947–69.
32. Jern P, Santtila P, Witting K, Alanko K, Harlaar N, Johansson A, et al. Premature and delayed ejaculation: genetic and environmental effects in a population-based sample of Finnish twins. J Sex Med. 2007;4(6):1739–49.
33. Morley JE, Haren MT, Kim MJ, Kevorkian R, Perry HM. Testosterone, aging and quality of life. J Endocrinol Invest. 2005;28(3 Suppl):76–80.
34. Carani C, Isidori AM, Granata A, Carosa E, Maggi M, Lenzi A, et al. Multicenter study on the prevalence of sexual symptoms in male hypo- and hyperthyroid patients. J Clin Endocrinol Metab. 2005;90(12):6472–9.
35. Bhasin S, Cunningham GR, Hayes FJ, Matsumoto AM, Snyder PJ, Swerdloff RS et al. Testosterone therapy in men with androgen deficiency syndromes: an Endocrine Society clinical practice guideline. J Clin Endocrinol Metab. 2010 Jun;95(6):2536–59.
36. Malkin CJ, Pugh PJ, Morris PD, Asif S, Jones TH, Channer KS. Low serum testosterone and increased mortality in men with coronary heart disease. Heart 2010;96(22):1821–25.
37. Li JY, Li XY, Li M, Zhang GK, Ma FL, Liu ZM, et al. Decline of serum levels of free testosterone in aging healthy Chinese men. Aging Male. 2005;8(3–4):203–6.
38. Shores MM, Matsumoto AM, Sloan KL, Kivlahan DR. Low serum testosterone and mortality in male veterans. Arch Intern Med. 2006;166(15):1660–5.
39. Wu FC, Tajar A, Beynon JM, Pye SR, Silman AJ, Finn JD et al. Identification of late-onset hypogonadism in middle-aged and elderly men. N Engl J Med. 2010;363(2):123–35.
40. Isidori AM, Giannetta E, Gianfrilli D, Greco EA, Bonifacio V, Aversa A, et al. Effects of testosterone on sexual function in men: results of a meta-analysis. Clin Endocrinol (Oxf). 2005;63(4):381–94.
41. Seftel A, Miner M, Kloner R, Althof S. Office evaluation of male sexual dysfunction. Urol Clin North Am. 2007;34(4):463–82.
42. Dennerstein L, Lehert P. Women's sexual functioning, lifestyle, mid-age, and menopause in 12 European countries. Menopause. 2004;11(6 Pt 2):778–85.
43. Rosen RC, Riley A, Wagner G, Osterloh IH, Kirkpatrick J, Mishra A. The international index of erectile function (IIEF): a multidimensional scale for assessment of erectile dysfunction. Urology. 1997;49(6):822–30.
44. Rosen RC, Cappelleri JC, Smith MD, Lipsky J, Peña BM. Development and evaluation of an abridged, 5-item version of the International Index of Erectile Function (IIEF-5) as a diagnostic tool for erectile dysfunction. Int J Impot Res. 1999;11(6):319–26.
45. Rosen RC, Catania JA, Althof SE, Pollack LM, O'Leary M, Seftel AD, et al. Development and validation of four-item version of Male Sexual Health Questionnaire to assess ejaculatory dysfunction. Urology. 2007;69(5):805–9.
46. Tancredi A, Reginster JY, Schleich F, Pire G, Maassen P, Luyckx F, et al. Interest of the androgen deficiency in aging males (ADAM) questionnaire for the identification of hypogonadism in elderly community-dwelling male volunteers. Eur J Endocrinol. 2004;151(3):355–60.
47. Daig I, Heinemann LA, Kim S, Leungwattanakij S, Badia X, Myon E, et al. The Aging Males' Symptoms (AMS) scale: review of its methodological characteristics. Health Qual Outcomes. 2003;1:77.
48. n RC, Araujo AB, Connor MK, Gerstenberger EP, Morgentaler A, Seftel AD, et al. The Hypogonadism Screener: psychometric validation in male patients and controls. Clin nol (Oxf). 2011;74(2):248–56.

49. Weissman MM, Sholomskas D, Pottenger M, et al. Assessing depressive symptoms in five psychiatric populations: a validation study. Am J Epidemiol. 1977;106(3):203–14.
50. Meston CM, Derogatis LR. Validated instruments for assessing female sexual function. J Sex Marital Ther. 2002;28 Suppl 1:155–64.
51. Wiegel M, Meston C, Rosen R. The female sexual function index (FSFI): cross-validation and development of clinical cutoff scores. J Sex Marital Ther. 2005;31(1):1–20.
52. Baser RE, Li Y, Carter J. Psychometric validation of the Female Sexual Function Index (FSFI) in cancer survivors. Cancer. 2012. doi: 10.1002/cncr.26739. [Epub ahead of print]
53. Gerstenberger EP, Rosen RC, Brewer JV, Meston CM, Brotto LA, Wiegel M, et al. Sexual desire and the female sexual function index (FSFI): a sexual desire cutpoint for clinical interpretation of the FSFI in women with and without hypoactive sexual desire disorder. J Sex Med. 2010;7(9):3096–103.
54. Kostis JB, Jackson G, Rosen R, Barrett-Connor E, Billups K, Burnett AL. Sexual dysfunction and cardiac risk (the Second Princeton Consensus Conference). Am J Cardiol. 2005;96(12B):85M–93.
55. Cardiometabolic Risks and Sexual Health: the Princeton III. November 8–10, 2010. Miami Beach, FL. Available from: http://cme.ouhsc.edu/documents/Course_11010_Princeton_reg_brochure.pdf.
56. Miner M, Esposito K, Guay A, Montorsi P, Goldstein I. Cardiometabolic risk and female sexual health: the Princeton III summary. J Sex Med. 2012;9(3):641–51; quiz 652.
57. Levine GN, Steinke EE, Bakaeen FG, Bozkurt B, Cheitlin MD, Conti JB et al. Sexual activity and cardiovascular disease: a scientific statement from the American Heart Association. Circulation. 2012 ;125(8):1058–72.
58. Impotence: NIH Consensus Development Panel on Impotence JAMA. 1993;270(1):83–90.
59. Seftel AD, Sun P, Swindle R. The prevalence of hypertension, hyperlipidemia, diabetes mellitus and depression in men with erectile dysfunction. J Urol. 2004;171(6):2341–5.
60. Miner M, Seftel AD. Centrally acting mechanisms for the treatment of male sexual dysfunction. Urol Clin North Am. 2007;34(4):483–96.
61. Lue TF. Erectile dysfunction. N Engl J Med. 2000;342:1802–13.
62. de Tejada IS, Goldstein I, Azadzoi K, Krane RJ, Cohen RA. Impaired neurogenic and endothelium-mediated relaxation of penile smooth muscle from diabetic men with impotence. N Engl J Med. 1989;320:1025–30.
63. Rajfer J, et al. Nitric oxide as a mediator of relaxation of the corpus cavernosum. N Engl J Med. 1992;326:1638.
64. Bancroft J. The endocrinology of sexual arousal. J Endocrinol. 2005;186:411–27.
65. Becker AJ, Uckert S, Stief CG, Scheller F, Knapp WH, Hartmann U, et al. Cavernous and systemic testosterone plasma levels during different penile conditions in healthy males and patients with erectile dysfunction. Urology. 2001;58(3):435–40.
66. Traish AM, Park K, Dhir V, Kim NN, Moreland RB, Goldstein I. Effects of castration and androgen replacement on erectile function in a rabbit model. Endocrinology. 1999;140(4):1861–8.
67. Zvara P, Sioufi R, Schipper HM, Begin LR, Brock GB. Nitric oxide mediated erectile activity is a testosterone dependent event: a rat erection model. Int J Impot Res. 1995;7(4):209–19.
68. Reilly CM, Lewis RW, Stopper VS, Mills TM. Androgenic maintenance of the rat erectile response via a non-nitric-oxide-dependent pathway. J Androl. 1997;18(6):588–94.
69. Hall R, Andrews PL, Hoyle CH. Effects of testosterone on neuromuscular transmission in rat isolated urinary bladder. Eur J Pharmacol. 2002;449(3):301–9.
70. Morley JE, Kaiser FE, Perry III HM, Patrick P, Morley PM, Stauber PM, et al. Longitudinal changes in testosterone, luteinizing hormone, and follicle-stimulating hormone in healthy older men. Metabolism. 1997;46(4):410–3.
71. Haren MT, Kim MJ, Tariq SH, Wittert GA, Morley JE. Andropause: a quality-of-life issue in older males. Med Clin North Am. 2006;90(5):1005–23.
72. Marcell TJ, Harman SM, Urban RJ, Metz DD, Rodgers BD, Blackman MR. Comparison of GH, IGF-I, and testosterone with mRNA of receptors and myostatin in skeletal muscle in older men. Am J Physiol Endocrinol Metab. 2001;281(6):E1159–64.

73. Benito M, Vasilic B, Wehrli FW, Bunker B, Wald M, Gomberg B, et al. Effect of testosterone replacement on trabecular architecture in hypogonadal men. J Bone Miner Res. 2005; 20(10):1785–91.
74. Dacal K, Sereika SM, Greenspan SL. Quality of life in prostate cancer patients taking androgen deprivation therapy. J Am Geriatr Soc. 2006;54(1):85–90.
75. Moffat SD, Zonderman AB, Metter EJ, Blackman MR, Harman SM, Resnick SM. Longitudinal assessment of serum free testosterone concentration predicts memory performance and cognitive status in elderly men. J Clin Endocrinol Metab. 2002;87(11): 5001–7.
76. Dunajska K, Milewicz A, Szymczak J, Jêdrzejuk D, Kuliczkowski W, Salomon P, et al. Evaluation of sex hormone levels and some metabolic factors in men with coronary atherosclerosis. Aging Male. 2004;7(3):197–204.
77. Muller M, van den Beld AW, Bots ML, Grobbee DE, Lamberts SW, van der Schouw YT. Endogenous sex hormones and progression of carotid atherosclerosis in elderly men. Circulation. 2004;109(17):2074–9.
78. English KM, Steeds RP, Jones TH, Diver MJ, Channer KS. Low-dose transdermal testosterone therapy improves angina threshold in men with chronic stable angina: A randomized, double-blind, placebo-controlled study. Circulation. 2000;102(16):1906–11.
79. Malkin CJ, Pugh PJ, Morris PD, Kerry KE, Jones RD, Jones TH, et al. Testosterone replacement in hypogonadal men with angina improves ischaemic threshold and quality of life. Heart. 2004;90(8):871–6.
80. Tsertsvadze A, Fink HA, Yazdi F, MacDonald R, Bella AJ, Ansari MT, et al. Oral phosphodiesterase-5 inhibitors and hormonal treatments for erectile dysfunction: a systematic review and meta-analysis. Ann Intern Med. 2009;151(9):650–61.
81. LeRoy TJ, Broderick GA. Doppler blood flow analysis of erectile function: who, when, and how. Urol Clin North Am. 2011;38(2):147–54.
82. Bhasin S, Cunningham GR, Hayes FJ. Testosterone therapy in men with androgen deficiency syndromes: an Endocrine Society clinical practice guideline. J Clin Endocrinol Metab. 2010;95:2536–59.
83. Vesper HW, Botelho JC, Shacklady C, et al. CDC project on standardizing steroid 380 hormone measurements. Steroids. 2008;73:1286–92.
84. Wang C, Nieschlag E, Swerdloff R, et al. Investigation, treatment, and monitoring of 385 late-onset hypogonadism in males: ISA, ISSAM, EAU, EAA, and ASA 386 recommendations. J Androl. 2009;30:1–9.
85. Institute of Medicine: Testosterone and aging: clinical research directions; 2003.
86. Psych Central. Psychology and Mental Heath News. Available from: http://psychcentral. com/news/2010/06/21/female-viagra-ineffective/14803.html.
87. Davis SR, Davison SL, Donath S, Bell RJ. Circulating androgen levels and self-reported sexual function in women. JAMA. 2005;294(1):91–6.
88. Wierman ME, Basson R, Davis SR, Khosla S, Miller KK, Rosner W, et al. Androgen therapy in women: an Endocrine Society Clinical Practice guideline. J Clin Endocrinol Metab. 2006;91(10):3697–710.
89. Amednews.com. Intrinsa stalled by concerns about safety. Available from: http://www.ama-assn.org/amednews/2005/01/17/hlsc0117.htm.
90. BioSante Pharmaceuticals. LibiGel product information. Available from: http://www.biosantepharma.com/LibiGel.php.
91. The Women's Health Initiative Participant Website. Conjugated equine estrogens and coronary heart disease. Available from: http://www.whi.org/findings/ht/ealone_chd.php.
92. Stefanick M, Anderson GL, Margolis KL, et al. Effects of conjugated equine estrogens on breast cancer and mammography screening in postmenopausal women with hysterectomy. JAMA. 2006;295(14):1647–57.
93. Buster JE. Transdermal menopausal hormone therapy: delivery through skin changes the rules. Expert Opin Pharmacother. 2010;11(9):1489–99.
94. Liebergall-Wischnitzer M, Paltiel O, Hochner Celnikier D, Lavy Y, Manor O, Woloski Wruble AC. Sexual function and quality of life of women with stress urinary incontinence:

a randomized controlled trial comparing the Paula Method (circular muscle exercises) to pelvic floor muscle training (PFMT) exercises. J Sex Med. 2012;9(6):1613–23.

95. Filocamo MT, Serati M, Frumenzio E, Li arzi V, Cattoni E, Champagne A, et al. The impact of mid-urethral slings for the treatment of urodynamic stress incontinence on female sexual function: a multicenter prospective study. J Sex Med. 2011;8(7):2002–8.

96. Goldstein I, Lue TF, Padma-Nathan H, Rosen RC, Steers WD, Wicker PA. Oral sildenafil in the treatment of erectile dysfunction. Sildenafil Study Group. N Engl J Med. 1998;338(20): 1397–404.

97. Brock GB, McMahon CG, Chen KK, Costigan T, Shen W, Watkins V, et al. Efficacy and safety of tadalafil for the treatment of erectile dysfunction: results of integrated analyses. J Urol. 2002;168(4 Pt 1):1332–6.

98. Hatzimouratidis K, Hatzichristou DG. Phosphodiesterase type 5 inhibitors: unmet needs. Curr Pharm Des. 2009;15(30):3476–85.

99. Fink HA, Mac Donald R, Rutks IR, Nelson DB, Wilt TJ. Sildenafil for male erectile dysfunction: a systematic review and meta-analysis. Arch Intern Med. 2002;162(12):1349–60.

100. Wagner G, Montorsi F, Auerbach S, Collins M. Sildenafil citrate (VIAGRA) improves erectile function in elderly patients with erectile dysfunction: a subgroup analysis. J Gerontol A Biol Sci Med Sci. 2001;56(2):M113–9.

101. Richter S, Vardi Y, Ringel A, Shalev M, Nissenkorn I. Intracavernous injections: still the gold standard for treatment of erectile dysfunction in elderly men. Int J Impot Res. 2001; 13(3):172–5.

102. Al-Najar A, Naumann CM, Kaufmann S, Steinbach-Jensch A, Hamann MF, Jünemann KP, et al. Should being aged over 70 years hinder penile prosthesis implantation? BJU Int. 2009; 104(6):834–7.

103. Conaglen HM, Conaglen JV. Investigating women's preference for sildenafil or tadalafil use by their partners with erectile dysfunction: the partners' preference study. J Sex Med. 2008; 5(5):1198–207.

104. Althof SE, Rubio-Aurioles E, Kingsberg S, Zeigler H, Wong DG, Burns P. Impact of tadalafil once daily in men with erectile dysfunction–including a report of the partners' evaluation. Urology. 2010;75(6):1358–63.

105. Rajfer J, Aliotta PJ, Steidle CP, Fitch III WP, Zhao Y, Yu A. Tadalafil dosed once a day in men with erectile dysfunction: a randomized, double-blind, placebo-controlled study in the US. Int J Impot Res. 2007;19(1):95–103.

106. Seftel AD, Buvat J, Althof SE, McMurray JG, Zeigler HL, Burns PR, et al. Improvements in confidence, sexual relationship and satisfaction measures: results of a randomized trial of tadalafil 5 mg taken once daily. Int J Impot Res. 2009;21(4):240–8.

107. Abrams P. Managing lower urinary tract symptoms in older men. Br Med J. 1995;310:1113–7.

108. Lepor H, Kazzazi A, Djavan B. α-Blockers for benign prostatic hyperplasia: the new era. Curr Opin Urol. 2012;22(1):7–15.

109. Braun M, Wassmer G, Klotz T, Reifenrath B, Mathers M, Engelmann U. Epidemiology of erectile dysfunction: results of the 'Cologne Male Survey'. Int J Impot Res. 2000;12(6): 305–11.

110. Rosen R, Altwein J, Boyle P, Kirby RS, Lukacs B, Meuleman E, et al. Lower urinary tract symptoms and male sexual dysfunction: the multinational survey of the aging male (MSAM-7). Eur Urol. 2003;44(6):637–49.

111. Mouli S, McVary KT. PDE5 inhibitors for LUTS. Prostate Cancer Prostatic Dis. 2009; 12(4):316–24.

112. Uckert S, Oelke M, Stief CG, Andersson KE, Jonas U, Hedlund P. Immunohistochemical distribution of cAMP- and cGMP-phosphodiesterase (PDE) isoenzymes in the human prostate. Eur Urol. 2006;49(4):740–5.

113. Morelli A, Filippi S, Mancina R, Luconi M, Vignozzi L, Marini M, et al. Androgens regulate phosphodiesterase type 5 expression and functional activity in corpora cavernosa. Endocrinology. 2004;145(5):2253–63.

114. Zhang X, Zang N, Wei Y, Yin J, Teng R, Seftel A. Testosterone regulates smooth muscle contractile pathways in the rat prostate: emphasis on PDE5 signaling. Am J Physiol Endocrinol Metab. 2012 Jan;302(2):E243-53. Epub 2011 Oct 25.
115. Uckert S, Sormes M, Kedia G, Scheller F, Knapp WH, Jonas U, et al. Effects of phosphodiesterase inhibitors on tension induced by norepinephrine and accumulation of cyclic nucleotides in isolated human prostatic tissue. Urology. 2008;71(3):526–30.
116. US Food and Drug Administration: news and events. FDA approves Cialis to treat benign prostatic hyperplasia. Available from: http://www.fda.gov/NewsEvents/Newsroom/PressAnnouncements/ucm274642.htm.
117. Oelke M, Giuliano F, Mirone V, Xu L, Cox D, Viktrup L. Monotherapy with tadalafil or tamsulosin similarly improved lower urinary tract symptoms suggestive of benign prostatic hyperplasia in an international, randomised, parallel, placebo-controlled clinical trial. Eur Urol. 2012;61(5):917–25.
118. Egerdie RB, Auerbach S, Roehrborn CG, Costa P, Garza MS, Esler AL, et al. Tadalafil 2.5 or 5 mg administered once daily for 12 weeks in men with both erectile dysfunction and signs and symptoms of benign prostatic hyperplasia: results of a randomized, placebo-controlled, double-blind study. J Sex Med. 2012;9(1):271–81.
119. Donatucci CF, Brock GB, Goldfischer ER, Pommerville PJ, Elion-Mboussa A, Kissel JD, et al. Tadalafil administered once daily for lower urinary tract symptoms secondary to benign prostatic hyperplasia: a 1-year, open-label extension study. BJU Int. 2011;107(7):1110–6.
120. McVary KT, Monnig W, Camps Jr JL, Young JM, Tseng LJ, van den Ende G. Sildenafil citrate improves erectile function and urinary symptoms in men with erectile dysfunction and lower urinary tract symptoms associated with benign prostatic hyperplasia: a randomized, double-blind trial. J Urol. 2007;177(3):1071–7.
121. Gacci M, Vittori G, Tosi N, Siena G, Rossetti MA, Lapini A, et al. A randomized, placebo-controlled study to assess safety and efficacy of vardenafil 10 mg and tamsulosin 0.4 mg vs. tamsulosin 0.4 mg alone in the treatment of lower urinary tract symptoms secondary to benign prostatic hyperplasia. J Sex Med. 2012;9(6):1624–33.
122. Lunenfeld B, Saad F, Hoesl CE. ISA, ISSAM and EAU recommendations for the investigation, treatment and monitoring of late-onset hypogonadism in males: scientific background and rationale. Aging Male. 2005;8(2):59–74.
123. Haren M, Chapman I, Coates P, Morley J, Wittert G. Effect of 12 month oral testosterone on testosterone deficiency symptoms in symptomatic elderly males with low-normal gonadal status. Age Ageing. 2005;34(2):125–30.
124. Kunelius P, Lukkarinen O, Hannuksela ML, Itkonen O, Tapanainen JS. The effects of transdermal dihydrotestosterone in the aging male: a prospective, randomized, double blind study. J Clin Endocrinol Metab. 2002;87(4):1467–72.
125. Shabsigh R. Testosterone therapy in erectile dysfunction and hypogonadism. J Sex Med. 2005;2(6):785–92.
126. Shabsigh R. Hypogonadism and erectile dysfunction: the role for testosterone therapy. Int J Impot Res. 2003;15 Suppl 4:S9–13.
127. Tariq SH, Haleem U, Omran ML, Kaiser FE, Perry III HM, Morley JE. Erectile dysfunction: etiology and treatment in young and old patients. Clin Geriatr Med. 2003;19(3):539–51.
128. Aversa A, Isidori AM, Spera G, Lenzi A, Fabbri A. Androgens improve cavernous vasodilation and response to sildenafil in patients with erectile dysfunction. Clin Endocrinol (Oxf). 2003;58(5):632–8.
129. Jain P, Rademaker AW, McVary KT. Testosterone supplementation for erectile dysfunction: results of a meta-analysis. J Urol. 2000;164(2):371–5.
130. Seftel AD, Mack RJ, Secrest AR, Smith TM. Restorative increases in serum testosterone levels are significantly correlated to improvements in sexual functioning. J Androl. 2004;25(6):963–72.
131. Testosterone topical solution (Axiron) for hypogonadism. Med Lett Drugs Ther. 2011 Jul 11;53(1368):54–5.

132. Kaufman JM, Miller MG, Fitzpatrick S, McWhirter C, Brennan JJ. One-year efficacy and safety study of a 1.62% testosterone gel in hypogonadal men: results of a 182-day open-label extension of a 6-month double-blind study. J Sex Med. 2012;9(4):1149–61.
133. Seftel A. Testosterone replacement therapy for male hypogonadism: part III. Pharmacologic and clinical profiles, monitoring, safety issues, and potential future agents. Int J Impot Res. 2007;19(1):2–24.
134. US Food and Drug Administration: drugs. Testosterone gel safety information. Available from: http://www.fda.gov/Drugs/DrugSafety/Postmarket Drug Safety Information for Patients and Providers/ucm161874.htm.
135. Morgentaler A. Testosterone and prostate cancer: what are the risks for middle-aged men? Urol Clin North Am. 2011;38(2):119–24.
136. Basaria S, Coviello A, Travison T, et al. Adverse events associated with testosterone administration. N Engl J Med. 2010;363:109–22.
137. Dandona P, Dhindsa S. Update: hypogonadotropic hypogonadism in type 2 diabetes and obesity. J Clin Endocrinol Metab. 2011;96(9):2643–51.
138. Corona G, Monami M, Rastrelli G, Aversa A, Tishova Y, Saad F, et al. Testosterone and metabolic syndrome: a meta-analysis study. J Sex Med. 2011;8(1):272–83.
139. Porst H. An overview of pharmacotherapy in premature ejaculation. J Sex Med. 2011;8 Suppl 4:335–41.
140. Melnik T, Althof S, Atallah AN, Puga ME, Glina S, Riera R. Psychosocial interventions for premature ejaculation. Cochrane Database Syst Rev. 2011;(8):CD008195.
141. McMahon CG. Dapoxetine for premature ejaculation. Expert Opin Pharmacother. 2010;11(10):1741–52.
142. AIDS Diagnoses by age. 2009. National center of health statistics. US Department of Health and Human Services Centers for Disease Control and Prevention. Available from: http://www.cdc.gov/hiv/topics/surveillance/basic.htm#aidsage.
143. AIDS among persons aged >50 years. Centers of Disease Control and Prevention, United States, 2009. Available from: http://www.cdc.gov/hiv/topics/over50/index.htm.
144. Senior K. Growing old with HIV. Lancet. 2005;5:739.
145. Wilson MM. Sexually transmitted diseases. Clin Geriatr Med. 2003;19:637–55.
146. Kaiser F. Sexual function and the older woman. Clin Geriatr Med. 2003;19(3):463–72.
147. Morley JE, Kaiser FE. Female sexuality. Med Clin North Am. 2003;87:1077–90.
148. Goetsch M. The effect of total hysterectomy on specific sexual sensations. Am J Obstet Gynecol. 2005;192:1922–7.
149. Johansson E, Steineck G, Holmberg L, Johansson JE, Nyberg T, Ruutu M, et al. Long-term quality-of-life outcomes after radical prostatectomy or watchful waiting: the Scandinavian Prostate Cancer Group-4 randomised trial. Lancet Oncol. 2011;12(9):891–9.
150. Anastasiou I, Yiannopoulou KG, Mihalakis A, Hatziandonakis N, Constantinides C. Symptoms of acute posttraumatic stress disorder in prostate cancer patients following radical prostatectomy. Am J Mens Health. 2011;5(1):84–9.
151. MacDonald R, Fink HA, Huckabay C, Monga M, Wilt TJ. Pelvic floor muscle training to improve urinary incontinence after radical prostatectomy: a systematic review of effectiveness. BJU Int. 2007;100(1):76–81.
152. Lee CT, Yeh CJ, Lee MC, Lin HS, Chen VC, Hsieh MH, et al. Leisure activity, mobility limitation and stress as modifiable risk factors for depressive symptoms in the elderly: results of a national longitudinal study. Arch Gerontol Geriatr. 2012;54(2):e221–9.
153. Kingsberg SA. The impact of aging on sexual function in women and their partners. Arch Sex Behav. 2002;31(5):431–7.
154. Kingsberg SA, Althof SE. Satisfying sexual events as outcome measures in clinical trial of female sexual dysfunction. J Sex Med. 2011;8(12):3262–70.

Index

T.J   et al. (eds.), *Primer of Geriatric Urology*, DOI 10.1007/978-1-4614-4773-3,   201
©   Science+Business Media New York 2013

Printed by Publishers' Graphics LLC